Doping and Public Policy

Doping and Public Policy

Edited by

John Hoberman and Verner Møller

University Press of Southern Denmark 2004

© The authors and University Press of Southern Denmark 2004
Printed by Narayana Press
ISBN: 87-7838-942-9
Cover design: Anne Charlotte Mouret
Cover illustration: Snapshot of illegal drug use. Photographed January 27, 1999.
Gorget Laurent/Corbis Sygma.

Published with support from:
The Danish Ministry of Culture

University Press of Southern Denmark
Campusvej 55
DK-5230 Odense M
Phone: +45 6615 7999
Fax: +45 6615 8126
Press@forlag.sdu.dk
www.universitypress.dk

Distribution in the United States and Canada:
International Specialized Book Services
5804 NE Hassalo Street
Portland, OR 97213-3644 USA
Phone: +1-800-944-6190
www.ibs.com

CONTENTS

INTRODUCTION
"DOPING AND PUBLIC POLICY"

John Hoberman

On 20 and 21 June 2002 an international group of specialists on doping in sport convened at the University of Southern Denmark (Odense) to participate in a conference on "Doping and Public Policy." The event was planned and carried out by the International Network for Humanistic Doping Research that is headquartered at the Institute of Sport Science and Clinical Biomechanics at the University of Southern Denmark. The volume now being published includes most of the papers that were delivered and discussed at the conference.

Most published work on the doping crisis in sport is based on the premise that the use of performance-enhancing drugs by elite or recreational athletes is both unethical and unhealthy, and the papers included in this volume generally conform to this perspective. The fact that the conference participants generally agree on the desirability of drug-free sport does not, however, mean that they are uncritical supporters of the anti-doping campaign that has been endorsed by many national and international sports federations and the International Olympic Committee. The purpose of the International Network for Humanistic Doping Research is to understand the doping phenomenon in its broadest cultural and political dimensions and to offer perspectives that may differ sharply from the standard anti-doping doctrine that underlies the official "War on Drugs" in elite sport. In this spirit, all of the speakers at the 2002 conference raised important questions about the global anti-doping campaign that are generally ignored by the sports officials and many of the journalists who together shape perceptions of the sports world that serves the emotional needs of many people around the world.

That the anti-doping campaign requires critical observers will be clear to anyone who has followed the doping-related public-relations disasters of the past twenty years. Indeed, the existence of this volume is one more sign that the campaign against doping drugs in elite sport has not gone well.[1] The widespread use of stimulants and synthetic hormone drugs such as anabolic steroids and the blood-booster erythropoietin (EPO) has produced an unending series of doping scandals in the high-performance sports world. Until recently, the two watershed events of this kind were the 1988 Ben Johnson scandal at the Seoul Olympic Games and the doping scandal that almost destroyed the 1998 Tour de France. The latest mega-scandal, the "designer steroid" (or BALCO) scandal that erupted in the United States in October 2003, appears to involve both Olympic athletes and American professionals who obtained drugs from a single

(American) source. The 2004 Athens Olympic Games, to be hosted by a government that has chosen to proclaim the innocence of its own doping suspects, is likely to be haunted by the doping issue like no other Olympiad that has preceded it.[2]

The doping epidemic in Olympic sport has flourished because for many years the IOC and the international sports federations affiliated with the Olympic movement did not develop or pursue a serious anti-doping strategy. The drug testing carried out by the IOC during the presidency of Juan Antonio Samaranch (1980-2001) was accompanied by many rhetorical assaults on the doping evil and was ineffective by any measure.[3] Drug testing at the Olympic Games between 1968 and 1996 produced a total of 52 positives for doping in an athlete population of about 54,000, or less than one per thousand.[4] The abolition of Olympic amateurism in 1981 created new incentives for doping by expanding the financial incentives for pursuing Olympic medals. Tightening Olympic qualifying norms further intensified the pressure on athletes to produce performances in any ways that they could to preserve their careers. The IOC Medical Commission, headed by the late Prince Alexandre de Merode, was widely seen as inept and ineffective. A well-known promoter of EPO-doping, Prof., Dr. Francesco Conconi, was hired in the early 1990s by the Medical Commission to develop a test for EPO and remains one of its members to this day.[5]

It was the 1998 Tour de France scandal that catalyzed the formation of the World Anti-Doping Agency (WADA) that began its operations in January 2000.[6] The establishment of WADA does represent, as **Barrie Houlihan** notes in his contribution to this volume, "a landmark in the development of [the] global anti-doping policy regime."[7] But how much can WADA actually do to anticipate, detect, deter, and punish athletes who are willing to engage in doping practices? Improvements in drug-detection technology have produced some successes, such as the surprise detections of Darbopoetin at the 2002 Salt Lake City Olympic Games and the "designer" anabolic steroid THG in late 2003. Yet we must also ask whether this approach to doping, or what **Ivan Waddington** calls the "conventional, punitive anti-doping framework," is the best way to deal with a doping problem that has so far proven to be intractable. Detect-and-punish has been standard procedure ever since the IOC introduced the drug testing of athletes in 1968. But is the virtually exclusive focus on the athlete who tests positive an adequate response to doping and its effects on both athletes and the millions of people who witness their performances?

Doping practices are embedded in a complex network of institutions and personal relationships that connect the athlete to many other actors in the doping system. Singling out the drug-consuming athlete for punishment and opprobrium has long served to divert attention away from the sports bureaucrats, politicians, and support personnel, including doctors, who benefit financially, politically, or emotionally from the doped performances of athletes who are held up for official condemnation when they are caught cheating. At this point, however, there is no sign that WADA intends to expand its anti-doping strategy beyond the search-and-sanction tactics that have been the standard operating procedure of anti-drug campaigns ever since the United

States government initiated its War on Drugs in 1909.[8] The papers collected in this volume suggest that the limitations of this strategy will inhibit the success of WADA for the foreseeable future. The possibility that genetic manipulation of athletes ("gene doping") will further complicate the anti-doping campaign is not addressed in this volume.

Analysis of the traditional doping control strategy can be done on three levels. On **the first (or "operational") level** one examines the specific anti-doping policies that are in place, determines how well they are being carried out, and proposes improvements that might make these measures more effective for catching doped athletes. Is unannounced testing carried out frequently enough to act as a deterrent to doping? Do doping control officers have the financial resources to track athletes to the often remote locations (South Africa, the Canary Islands, the Bahamas) they have found so congenial for training purposes? Do sports federations have the financial resources and legal expertise to engage in lawsuits with athletes who have tested positive for doping drugs? Why have the appeals boards of so many national and even international federations around the world exonerated athletes charged with doping offences?[9] Do such cases result from inadequate disciplinary codes or biased rulings that originate in nationalistic sentiments among those adjudicating these cases? And are the tests themselves scientifically valid? In 2003 it was discovered that the standard test for EPO, which requires days of laboratory work and is very expensive, was flawed. A urine sample submitted by the Kenyan runner Bernard Lagat in August 2003, first analysed as a positive and then as a negative, demonstrated, as one German scientist put it, "a chemical profile that has never been seen before. We simply do not know what is going on." Werner Franke, the German cell biologist and anti-doping activist commented: "The worst thing that can happen to the anti-doping campaign is unreliable testing procedures."[10]

Operational problems can also result from bureaucratic disagreements about how to categorize the use of specific drugs. For example, when the Spanish cyclist Igor Gonzalez de Galdeano tested positive for the asthma medication Salbutamol during the 2002 Tour de France, both the Société du Tour de France and the International Cycling Union (UCI) refused to classify this as a doping offence because the drug had been registered in the rider's health passport, and despite the fact that his reading of 1360 nanograms per milliliter exceeded the maximum allowable limit of 1000 ng/ml. "Igor is sick," said the chief of the Once team, "he suffers from asthma, as I do, and he will have to use an inhaler for as long as he lives. That is a health problem and not doping." But Dr. Alain Garnier, director of WADA's European office, judged Galdeano's Salbutamol level to be "extremely rare and even extraordinary." "This reading cannot be explained as a normal therapeutic intervention," he said. The French anti-doping agency (CPLD) sided with WADA. The Tour director, Daniel Baal, spoke regretfully of "a conflict among experts where there are different interpretations." In March 2003, WADA, the CPLD, and the UCI agreed on a six-month ban that excluded the rider from the 2003 Tour and marked a policy defeat for the UCI, which continues to publicize its disagreements with WADA.[11]

Such conflicts between federations and agencies are a major structural feature of an international sports system that attempts to reconcile international standards and agreements with the self-defined needs of national bodies that are responsible for producing medal-winning performances in international competitions. The Salbutamol case also demonstrated how the eroding boundary between therapeutic and performance-enhancing procedures can complicate the defining and adjudicating of a certain class of doping cases. Despite such complications, however, the operational level of analysis assumes that adequate funding and proper administration of this network of institutions and federations can result in a truly effective anti-doping arrangement that will detect and punish doping athletes and deter potential violators of the anti-doping code.

The second (or "structural") level of analysis takes a less optimistic view of this anti-doping "arrangement" for two reasons. First, it does not take for granted the integrity or the competence of the various bodies that constitute the anti-doping system. Given their long record of ineffectiveness, the anti-doping programs of bodies such as the IOC and the national and international federations (as well as their respective medical commissions) should be appraised skeptically rather than credulously. For one thing, the motivations of those who aspire to leadership roles in sports federations may be incompatible with a serious and honest commitment to anti-doping work.[12] Second, the "structural" analysis sees this anti-doping "arrangement" as embedded in the larger sociopolitical context that includes nationalist politicians and commercial interests such as pharmaceutical companies, as well as the global black market for doping drugs that have been diverted from the legitimate distribution network that serves medical needs.[13]

Both aspects of the "structural" approach to the anti-doping system are addressed by **Alessandro Donati** in his contribution to this volume. In the course of his long, distinguished, and sometimes dangerous career as Italy's foremost anti-doping activist, Donati exposed and pursued key players in Italy's sports-political complex, a virtual *Who's Who* of the corrupt political elite that ran Italian sport at the national level for many years. The late Primo Nebiolo, who was inducted into the IOC in 1994, served as president of the International Association of Athletics Federation (IAAF) for almost two decades (1981-1999) and was implicated in the long-jump cheating scandal at the 1987 IAAF Athletics Championships in Rome. Dr. Francesco Conconi, whose blood doping activities were exposed in the Swedish press as early as 1985[14], kept Nebiolo informed about his secret use of EPO with many elite athletes.[15] Conconi was financed by Mario Pescante, president of the Italian Olympic Committee (CONI), who lost this position in 1998 on account of the corruption scandal that closed the CONI doping laboratory at Acqua Acetosa near Rome.[16] Pescante retained his position on the IOC and was made minister of sport by Silvio Berlusconi after his election as prime minister in 2001. (Berlusconi dismissed the CONI lab scandal as a left-wing conspiracy against the honor of Italian sport.[17]) Pescante ignored the report on Italian doping practices Donati gave him in 1993. Three years later Donati provided this report to the UCI, which instituted hematocrit surveillance as a form of doping control in early 1997. Conconi spent years on trial for offenses against Italy's anti-doping law. In November 2003 he was acquitted by a judge because the statute of limitations had passed. In March 2004 a judge in Ferrera pronounced Conconi guilty of having aided and abetted in the EPO doping of many athletes.[18] Conconi remains to this day Vice Rector of the University of Ferrera and, remarkably, spent many years as a member of both the IOC and UCI medical commissions.

Structural analysis of this Italian scenario focuses on the network that conjoins political figures and sports officials as well as the sportive nationalist uses to which this network can be put. It must also assess the balance of power between these actors and the Italian state prosecutors and judges who have been Donati's allies in the struggle against the doping subculture. Structural analysis requires, in other words, a political sociology of the doping system and its adversaries that describes the relevant interest groups, conflicts and alliances. During the Berlusconi period, Italian sportive nationalism has operated from the very top of the political system. Prime Minister Berlusconi is the owner of the successful AC Milan professional football club and has integrated sportive themes into his political campaigns. His claim in 2001 that "all the talk about doping" in Italian sport was no more than "a plot by the political left" is an extreme example of the sportive nationalist demagoguery that other politicians have employed against suspicions that the nation's athletic heroes practice doping.[19] For example, Prime Minister John Howard made a point of defending the reputation of his nation's athletes in 2001 during a scandal involving an Australian Institute of Sport swim coach. "I want you to know," he wrote to one swimming star, "that you and the entire Australian swim team has [sic] the support and respect of myself and the nation."[20] When the sprinter Merlene Ottey tested positive for nandrolone in 1999, the President of Jamaica and his Minister for Sport and Labor supported her.[21] In February 2004 the Greek sports minister, Giorgio Lianos, defended the nation's star sprinters against longstanding suspicions that they were involved in doping. His proud declaration that these athletes had "never tested positive" came only six months before the scheduled opening of the Athens Olympic Games.[22] Given the willingness of politicians to play on this theme, it is not surprising that in 2002 the Italian cycling star Marco Pantani called on Prime Minister Berlusconi to speak out against what he called the "persistent and unwarranted suspicions and slanders" being directed at professional cyclists.[23] In summary, sportive nationalism in its various forms has subverted the anti-doping campaign often and in many countries around the world.

Several participants in the conference have made significant contributions to the structural analysis of doping. Hans B. Skaset leaves us with no illusions about the lack of interest in doping control he has encountered at the highest levels of sports administration. Indeed, his own career is an illustration of the imbalance of power that has usually left anti-doping reformers at a disadvantage vis-à-vis sportive nationalists. Following a controversy involving two Norwegian athletes at the Sydney Olympic Games, his principled position against "gray zone" practices such as the use of altitude chambers and supplements forced his resignation from the Norwegian Ministry of Culture in October 2000.[24]

The structural analysis of the doping system is exemplified by the work of **Karl-Heinrich Bette**. His sociological writings describe in impressive detail the social structure of the doping subculture that benefits interest groups that are seldom called to account for their roles in the doping crisis, even as athletes are subject to public accusation and professional ruin.[25] Doping penalties imposed on individuals offer the public a never-ending soap opera that covers up the *systemic* character of the doping phenomenon. Bette argues that "contrary to some familiar and premature judgments, doping is not something that can simply be traced back to the personality traits of individual athletes, coaches, officials or sports physicians. Doping is less a case of 'bad' people than of social conditions that produce deviance in predictable ways. As a sociologist, one might well ask, how is it that elite sport has brought together such an assortment of actors, irrespective of discipline or nationality, that collectively demonstrates so many character flaws?" This observation should give pause to those who claim that elite athletes are worthy role models for young people, since the enforcement of doping rules produces an unending stream of elite athletes who have ostensibly disgraced themselves before the eyes of the world. For this very reason, proponents of the role-modeling argument should support the structural analysis of doping as a strategy that can explain this deviant behavior as something other than the result of ethically defective personalities that may be beyond redemption. Indeed, the most radical of Bette's propositions is the substitution of sociological analysis for the moral outrage and condemnation that have become a standard feature of anti-doping rhetoric. For those who promote elite athletes as moral exemplars have somehow overlooked the merciless and life-distorting demands on high-performance athletes that produce what Bette calls "the compatibility of deviance and the logic of elite sport."

Structural analysis offers in addition a variety of critical observations about the distorted relationships that develop within the high-performance sports milieu. **Andreas Singler and Gerhard Treutlein** criticize the authoritarian approach of the coaching profession and in particular the dependency relationships that develop between male coaches and female athletes who are "enticed" into doping.[26] "The aim of coaches," they write, "should be to slowly loosen the ties with their athletes and make themselves superfluous." This egalitarian principle directly challenges the paternalism of the coaching profession and the domination-submission model it so often promotes.

So-called "educational" strategies against doping that are designed as a form of moral instruction are a symptom of this paternalism. "Experience teaches us," they report, "that talking about ethics and social and educational objectives generally gets you nowhere." Coaches whose jobs depend on their getting the best performances out of their athletes are in no position to address the existential issues that are the core of any real moral education. In these relationships paternalism and authoritarianism displace the genuine moral instruction that would discredit the performance principle as the ultimate objective of sport. Like Singler and Treutlein, the French physician and anti-doping activist **Patrick Laure** argues that doping prevention is a complex process that is incompatible with subordinating the lives of young athletes to the pursuit of sheer performance. Subjecting people to the Darwinian demands of elite sport does not promote the kind of self-esteem that is rooted in ethical reflection. The simplistic use of scare tactics to dissuade young people from using drugs is guaranteed to fail. Laure's essay is a pointed reminder of the profound limitations associated with taking a "War on Drugs" approach to the prevention of doping behavior.

In fact, anti-doping "education" has been a familiar policy of institutions, such as the IOC and the United States Olympic Committee (USOC), that long ago forfeited their credibility vis-à-vis anti-doping efforts. This kind of "education" has served instead as a fig leaf that is meant to conceal the unscrupulous pragmatism of the medal-winning machines. Following the doping scandal that devastated elite cross-country skiing in Finland in February 2001, the Finnish Skiing Association (FSA) introduced an educational program of this kind.[27] Less than three years later another doping scandal demonstrated that this program had failed, at which point the FSA general secretary, Jari Piirainen, offered the following advice to his foreign colleagues: "Don't be too naïve."[28]

For more than a century, high-performance sport has been what the German sports physician Wildor Hollmann has called "a gigantic experiment carried out on the human organism."[29] **Giselher Spitzer**, the leading expert on the East German doping system and a prominent defender of its victims, shows how this experiment mutated into a bizarre and criminal enterprise in the former German Democratic Republic.[30] With its own pharmaceutical company (Jenapharm) and a small army of willing doctors and scientists, State Plan 14.25 transformed the inherent logic of high-performance sport into the most extreme version of sportive nationalism the world has ever known.

At the same time, it is important to understand that East German sports medicine was essentially a caricature of the increasingly aggressive sports medicine that is embraced by physicians and elite athletes in many societies.[31] It is both easy and misleading to think of the old East German sports system as a kind of gulag for athletes whose purposes and methods were fundamentally alien to our own system of values. In fact, they were not, as the Finns discovered in 2001 when they found themselves comparing their own sport culture to that of the old GDR.[32] It turned out that some of their "legendary" cross-country skiers found doping as natural as their East German counterparts had done back in the 1980s. The head of the IAAF Medical Commission, Arne Ljungqvist, announced that he was "shocked" to find an entire cabal of doctors and coaches colluding (GDR-style) in a doping scheme.[33] On the other side of the Atlantic, the same mentality prevails. The so-called Oregon Project (sponsored by Nike) that aims at producing American marathon runners who can compete with the Africans is an almost comical attempt to mimic the obsessive and manipulative techniques of the East Germans.[34] The miserable failure of the German athletics team at the IAAF World Championships in Paris in August 2003 prompted one Social Democratic politician, Peter Danckert, to call for a return to the old GDR model that had worked so well before 1989.[35] The problem with this proposal, as Thomas Kistner noted at the time, was that the old GDR system had employed a pharmacological regimen that was now politically incorrect.[36]

⧫ A major cause of our own doping problem is the unwillingness of sports officials and others to openly acknowledge the often brutal demands of high-performance sport and the often unattractive medical consequences of subjecting athletes to these ordeals. As Bette points out, today's elite athletes need comprehensive support systems simply to function in an environment where only the fit survive and where most of the competitors wind up as losers. **Verner Møller's** contribution to this volume represents what we may call **the "radical" level of analysis** that calls into question some of the basic premises of the anti-doping campaign.[37] His role is to examine some of the awkward questions that are routinely ignored by those who are working to eliminate drugs from sport.

Møller's fundamental argument is that anti-doping campaigners have failed to grasp the thoroughly amoral essence of high-performance sport. The sportive contests that really matter to enormous audiences around the world are dramatic spectacles whose value is entirely aesthetic and not the least bit moral. What counts is willpower rather than ethics; the elite athlete's code of conduct is an ethos that is meant to sharpen the confrontation between rivals whose only obligation is to the drama of the spectacle itself. What is more, no one who is aware of the medical costs of elite sport will endorse the idea that it promotes good health. On the contrary, what sport offers is "intoxicating experiences that involve presence, excitement and an uncompromising devotion that puts health at risk." As the boxing fan Bertolt Brecht once put it: "Great sport begins where good health ends."[38] In summary, Møller argues, elite sport is irrelevant to the promotion of either health or virtue.

The anti-doping campaign is an exercise in social engineering that assumes precisely the opposite, namely, that elite athletes have a legitimate function as character-building role models for the larger society. The drug testing that Møller objects to as an unwarranted invasion of privacy is intended to deter socially undesirable behavior that would allegedly proliferate throughout the masses if it were tolerated in popular athletes. But this line of thinking typically evades three important questions. First, what is the pedagogical value of exemplary behaviour that requires policing and the threat of punishment to produce it? As of November 2001, the hematocrits of Finnish cross-country skiers were being posted on the Internet.[39] Yet one wonders how many people actually took the trouble to monitor the red blood cell counts of their favorite athletes. Second, are anti-drug activists really unaware that enormous numbers of people, including young people, have already lost their innocence regarding the performance-enhancing drugs that are now a part of everyday life both inside and outside the world of sport? According to the Centre National de la Recherche Scientifique (CNRS) in Paris, most young children in France already believe that performance-enhancing drugs belong in sport: "Children of six years find it just as legitimate to take drugs to improve sporting performance as it is to take them to cure a sickness," according to the professor who supervised the survey.[40] Third, is it not fraudulent to speak of a "drug-free" sport that both allows and encourages athletes to stuff themselves with "supplements" and other substances that are not on the prohibited list of doping substances? It would be more accurate to speak of "hormone-free" sport, although even this standard is breached by the UCI, which allows its cyclists to boost their hematocrit levels to 49% with EPO or in any other way they can manage it. It is also worth keeping in mind that the IOC that claims to want "drug-free" sport today once administered a drug testing program that, between 1968 and 1996, identified every thousandth athlete as a doping violator.[41] (This astonishingly ineffective record is currently being matched by the United States Anti-Doping Agency.[42]) Now let us think about how much WADA can do to produce a different result.

Møller's analysis is bad news for the anti-doping campaign because it demonstrates once again that the only really compelling argument against doping is essentially intuitive. This is not an original observation; as Sir Arthur Porritt put it in 1965: "To define doping is, if not impossible, at best extremely difficult, and yet everyone who takes part in competitive sport or who administers it knows exactly what it means. The definition lies not in words but in integrity of character."[43] Møller's accomplishment has been to explore the consequences of this situation with more rigor than those who have preceded him. In fact, careful examination of the various arguments that have been cobbled together to form the standard case against doping does reveal a weak structure that has been effectively obscured by the (intuitive) moral certainty that doping is simply wrong.

The major weakness of the anti-doping campaign is not to be found in the laboratories that try to detect illicit drugs. It is rather that the campaigners refuse to confront honestly some of the facts of life about doping that shape the real world in which elite athletes pursue their careers. First, the very idea of "drug-free" sport is a puritanical fiction; pharmacological support has been an integral part of high-performance sport since the 1890s. Elite athletes have long felt entitled to use drugs[44], and today they consume massive quantities of "supplements," vitamins, and various medications.[45] The UCI allowed the doctors treating the Tour de France riders in 2001 to use as many as 300 drugs for this purpose, and then refused to publish the list.[46] Second, public demand for "drug-free" sport is diminishing as the use of performance-enhancing drugs by the general public is increasing. Surveys published in late 2003 in the United States show that a quarter of those questioned already accept the medically regulated use of doping drugs by professional athletes.[47] Third, imposing Olympic-style doping penalties on athlete-workers (such as cyclists) is incompatible with sport as a commercial enterprise. This fact accounts for the longstanding feud between WADA and the UCI. As the UCI website puts it: "A two-year ban is too harsh if, for example, it puts a de facto end to an athlete's career." WADA's willingness to negotiate penalties with the UCI and FIFA thus acknowledges the long tradition that allows professional athletes to use doping drugs.

Finally, the hygienic paternalism that denies athletes doping drugs on the grounds that they are dangerous to health offers too selective a list of health issues to be credible. Real concern for the health of professional athletes takes the form of serious public health research and legally compelled testimony, as exemplified by the investigations of the Italian state prosecutor Raffaele Guariniello.[48] The UCI's hematocrit testing, while medically useful, is dilettantish by comparison, because the UCI and the judge from Turin have different goals. Guariniello is a specialist in occupational diseases who takes a comprehensive approach to the medical well-being of professional athletes, while Hein Verbruggen of the UCI is, in effect, a union boss who is looking out primarily for his athletes' economic well-being. As an academic expert on health, Møller understands the absurdity of pretending that the reparative sports medicine of the Tour or professional soccer has anything to do with the medicine that aims to preserve and enhance human health. Nor is he particularly alarmed by this discrepancy, since he endorses the athlete's right to engage in whatever physiological adventure the athlete chooses to embrace. What he does object to is the improbable idea that elite sport can be tamed by hygiene.

Notes

1   For a chronology of doping control in elite sport, see Jan Todd and Terry Todd, "Significant Events in the History of Drug Testing and the Olympic Movement, 1960-1999," in Wayne Wilson and Edward Derse, eds., *Doping in Elite Sport: The Politics of Drugs in the Olympic Movement* (Champaign, IL: Human Kinetics, 2001): 65-128.

2   In February 2004, the Greek sports minister, Giorgio Lianos, attempted to refute an allegation that tied the prominent Greek coach of the nation's sprinting stars to the "designer steroid" scandal that had erupted in the United States in October 2003. Lianos denounced "anti-Greek propaganda that defames and insults Greek sport." Only six months before the opening of the 2004 Athens Olympics, Lianos was offering a somewhat histrionic defense of what he called "the credibility of the Greek athletes, their coaches and the credibility of the Olympic Games." See "Greek coach says he will sue British newspaper," Associated Press (February 18, 2004).). The Greek sprinting stars who have been widely suspected of doping are Kostas Kenteris and Ekaterina Thanou. See "Pfiffe des Zweifels," *Süddeutsche Zeitung* (August 12, 2002); "Der undurchsichtige Adonis," *Der Spiegel* (August 11, 2003): 87.

3   See, for example, John Hoberman, "How Drug Testing Fails: The Politics of Doping Control," in Wayne Wilson and Edward Derse, eds., *Doping in Elite Sport: The Politics of Drugs in the Olympic Movement* (Champaign, IL: Human Kinetics, 2001): 241-274.

4   See Amy Shipley, "Drug Tests, Troubling Results: IOC's System Is Plagued by False Positives in Addition to Cheating," *Washington Post* (September 23, 1999); Amy Shipley, "With Drug Tests, Answers Are Few: The IOC Says It Is Cracking Down on Doping, But to Critics the Problem Is Only Getting Worse," *Washington Post* (September 22, 1999).

5   See "Moralisch schuldig," *Süddeutsche Zeitung* (March 12, 2004); "Ein belastender Freispruch Conconis," *Neue Zürcher Zeitung* (March 13, 2004). On Conconi's career as a promoter of doping, see Hoberman, "How Drug Testing Fails: The Politics of Doping Control," 251-252.

6   See Jim Ferstle, "World Conference on Doping in Sport," in Wayne Wilson and Edward Derse, eds., *Doping in Elite Sport: The Politics of Drugs in the Olympic Movement* (Champaign, IL: Human Kinetics, 2001): 275-286.

7   See, for example, Barrie Houlihan, *Dying to win. Doping in sport and the development of anti-doping policy* (Strasbourg: Council of Europe Publishing, 1999).

8   "The social use of cocaine by underworld characters and delinquent young men going through the stresses of adolescence began the transformation of our view of drug-users from eccentrics with a specialised vice into evil criminals and menacing enemies of society. The US Opium Exclusion Act of 1909 began diverting drug-users from the more innocuous opium-smoking to the more destructive intravenous use of heroin. The US Harrison Narcotic Act of 1914 provided the model for drug prohibi-

tion legislation throughout the Western World." See Richard Davenport-Hines, *The Pursuit of Oblivion: A Global History of Narcotics* (New York and London: W.W. Norton & Company, 2002): 14.

9   One limitation of the system that imposes doping sanctions concerns the level at which a drug must be present to qualify as a positive. For example, in 2003 Carl Lewis and seven other American athletes were exonerated by the international track and field federation (IAAF) for having tested positive in 1988 for levels of stimulants that fell below the standard that defines a doping offence. See "Mehr Zweifel," *Süddeutsche Zeitung* (May 2, 2003).

10   "Die Schrecken der Abschreckung," *Süddeutsche Zeitung* (October 4/5, 2003).

11   See "Asthmatiker im Zwielicht," *Süddeutsche Zeitung* (July 19, 2002); "Galdeano gesperrt," *Süddeutsche Zeitung* (May 2, 2003).

12   See Hoberman, "How Drug Testing Fails: The Politics of Doping Control," 241-274.

13   The Böhringer pharmaceutical company supplied the EPO Conconi injected into his stable of elite athletes, who included Manuela di Centa, who is now a member of the IOC. See "Ein belastender Freispruch Conconis," *Neue Zürcher Zeitung* (March 15, 2004).

14   "'Professorn' bakom det italienska undret," *Svenska Dagbladet* (March 11, 1985).

15   Interview with Sandro Donati in "Doping – ein kollektiver Wahnsinn," *Neue Zürcher Zeitung* (March 25, 2000).

16   "Liebesgrüße aus dem Heizungskeller," *Süddeutsche Zeitung* (October 19, 1998).

17   "Klagen über geschäftsschädigende Kontrollen," *Süddeutsche Zeitung* (April 24, 2001).

18   "Moralisch schuldig," *Süddeutsche Zeitung* (March 12, 2004).

19   "Der Vorkämpfer," *Der Spiegel* (March 4, 2002): 230.

20   "Australia's swimming in scandal," *The Guardian* (April 16, 2001).

21   "Denken diese Leute, wir sind Idioten?" *Süddeutsche Zeitung* (August 20, 1999).

22   "Greek coach says he will sue British newspaper," Associated Press (February 18, 2004).

23   "Pirat am seidenen Faden," *Süddeutsche Zeitung* (May 4/5, 2002).

24   See, for example, "Truer med å trekke offentlig støtte," *Aftenposten* (October 27, 2000); »Full seier til Kran,« *Aftenposten* (October 28, 2000).

25   See, for example, Karl-Heinrich Bette and Uwe Schimank, *Doping im Hochleistungssport* (Frankfurt am Main: Suhrkamp, 1995).

26   See, for example, Andreas Singler and Gerhard Treutlein, *Doping im Spitzensport: Sportwissenschaftliche Analysen zur nationalen und internationalen Leistungsentwicklung* (Aachen: Myer & Meyer Verlag, 2000).

27   "Erste Regung nach dem großen Crash," *Suddeutsche Zeitung* (November 24/25, 2001).

28   "Rückkehr der bösen Gedanken," *Süddeutsche Zeitung* (November 29/30, 2003).

29   W[ildor] Hollmann, "Risikofaktoren in der Entwicklung des Hochleistungssports," in H. Rieckert, ed., *Sportmedizin-Kursbestimmung* [Deutscher Sportärztekongreß, Kiel, 16.-19. Oktober 19860 (Berlin: Springer Verlag, 1987): 15.

30   See, for example, Giselher Spitzer, *Doping in der DDR: Ein historischer Überblick zu einer konspirativen Praxis* (Cologne: Sport und Buch, 2000).

31   See, for example, Ivan Waddington, *Sport, Health and Drugs: A Critical Sociological Perspective* (London and New York: E & FN Spon, 2000); John Hoberman, "Sports Physicians and the Doping Crisis in Elite Sport," *Clinical Journal of Sport Medicine* 12 (2002): 203-208.

32   "Die Johnsons aus Finnland," *Süddeutsche Zeitung* (March 2, 2001).

33   Thomas Hahn, "Das Herz eines Langläufers," *Süddeutsche Zeitung* (March 8, 2001).

34   See Andrew Tilin, "The Ultimate Running Machine, *Wired Magazine* (August 2002).

35   "Loblied auf DDR-Sport," *Süddeutsche Zeitung* (September 13/14, 2003).

36   Thomas Kistner, "Vorwärts in die Vergangenheit," *Süddeutsche Zeitung* (September 13/14, 2003).

37   See Møller's polemical study *Dopingdjævlen* [*The Doping Devil*] (Copenhagen: Gyldendal, 1999). On the reaction in Denmark to its publication see John Hoberman, "The Reception of *Dopingdjævlen* (1999) in Denmark," in Jørn Hansen and Thomas Skovgaard, eds., *Sportens væsen og uvæsen* (Odense: Syddansk Universitetsforlag, 2002): 133-140.

38 "Der große Sport fängt da an, wo er längst aufgehört hat, gesund zu sein."

39 "Erste Regung nach dem großen Crash," *Süddeutsche Zeitung* (November 24/25, 2001).

40 "French children regard doping as normal," Associated Press (March 24, 2004).

41 See Amy Shipley, "Drug Tests, Troubling Results: IOC's System Is Plagued by False Positives in Addition to Cheating," *Washington Post* (September 23, 1999); Amy Shipley, "With Drug Tests, Answers Are Few: The IOC Says It Is Cracking Down on Doping, But to Critics the Problem Is Only Getting Worse," *Washington Post* (September 22, 1999).

42 "In 2003, the United States Anti-Doping Agency conducted 6,890 drug tests. Only six (0.09 percent) were positive. These results do not measure the use of performance-enhancing strategies for which no tests are currently available." See Charles Yesalis and Michael Bahrke, "Where There Is a Will to Gain an Edge, Athletes Find a Way," *New York Times* (March 7, 2004).

43 At the time Porritt was the chairman of the British Association of Sports Medicine. See "Doping," *The Journal of Sports Medicine and Physical Fitness* 5 (1965): 166; quoted in *Commission of Inquiry into the Use of Drugs and Banned Practices Intended to Increase Athletic Performance* (Ottawa: Canadian Government Publishing Centre, 1990): 77-78.

44 "There was no centralized drug testing at the 1964 [Olympic] Games in Tokyo; some spot checks were done but many athletes refused to cooperate with the [IOC] medical commission." See "State-of-the-Art Drug Identification Laboratories Play Increasing Role in Major Athletic Events," *Journal of the American Medical Association* 256 (December 12, 1996): 3073.

45 See, for example, Christopher Clarey, "The Unnatural World of Legal Performance Aids," *International Herald Tribune* (October 3, 2003); "Happy Hour: Cocktails machen die Beine schnell," *Neue Zürcher Zeitung* (October 5, 2003).

46 "Tour-medicinmænd," *Information* (June 22, 2001).

47 See Bill Briggs, "Swifter, Higher, Stronger, Dirtier?" *Denver Post* (November 16, 2003); Jere Longman and Marjorie Connelly, "Americans Suspect Steroid Use In Sports Is Common, Poll Finds," *New York Times* (December 16, 2003). For additional commentary on the American public's indifference to doped professional baseball players, see Tom Verducci, "Totally Juiced," *Sports Illustrated* (June 3, 2002): 48.

48 See, for example, "Dafür sorgen, daß Doping geächtet wird," *Süddeutsche Zeitung* (May 5, 1999); "Der Vorkämpfer," Der Spiegel (March 4, 2002): 228-230.

CHAPTER 1

HARMONISING ANTI-DOPING POLICY: THE ROLE OF THE WORLD ANTI-DOPING AGENCY

Barrie Houlihan

From the late 1980s it has generally been acknowledged that the problem of doping in sport has outgrown the scope and powers of domestic public anti-doping authorities and was testing, to the limit, the capacity of international and national sports federations. The greater geographical mobility of athletes, the rapid commercialisation of a number of sports, the increased sophistication of new drugs and doping techniques and, above all, the growing litigiousness of athletes were changes in the environment of anti-doping policy which added urgency to the development of an effective global anti-doping policy regime.

Krasner has defined a policy regime as principles, norms, rules and decision-making procedures around which actor expectations converge in a given issue-area (Krasner 1983: 1). "Principles are beliefs of fact, causation, and rectitude. Norms are standards of behavior defined in terms of rights and obligations. Rules are specific prescriptions or proscriptions for action. Decision-making procedures are prevailing practices for making and implementing collective choice" (Krasner 1983: 2). Given the scope of this definition, regimes might be articulated in formal legal instruments with a secretariat and other supporting formal institutions, while others may exist only as a set of shared expectations among policy actors and lack any significant organisational component. Table 1 identifies the most common characteristics of well established regimes and shows that prior to the formation of the World Anti-Doping Agency (WADA) the anti-doping policy regime was weak, both in terms of the clarity of its principles, its norms, and in terms of its organisational infrastructure. The anti-doping regime prior to 1999 was characterised by fragmentation of effort, mutual suspicion among key actors, a general lack of momentum and a severe lack of resources. While there was much activity, there was little effective action.

Table 1: The anti-doping regime prior to the establishment of WADA in 1999.

Characteristic	The anti-doping regime prior to the establishment of WADA
A degree of stability in the pattern of relations between core actors.	A stable, but poorly co-ordinated, group of policy actors which included the IOC, the major Olympic international federations (IFs), the Council of Europe and a small number of "activist" governments.
A process by which some interests emerge as core actors and others are marginalised.	The scope of participation in policy discussion was largely determined, for sports organisations, by acceptance onto the Olympic programme and, for states, by participation in the work of the Council of Europe or membership of regional groupings of states (e.g. International Anti-Doping Arrangement) The IOC, the major federations and activist states emerged as core actors often as a result of scandal, external pressure or fear that other actors would intervene and determine a policy response which would be to their disadvantage. However, it is notable that the voice of athletes, though often referred to, had no formal independent representation.
Key functions of regime maintenance are fulfilled by a permanent secretariat or an agreed division of labour between key actors and include policy review and the monitoring, verification and, in some regimes, the enforcement of compliance.	Fulfilled only weakly and in an unsystematic fashion. Occasional conferences to exchange information and experience and to debate policy. Policy debates tended to take place in two parallel arenas, one focused on the IOC and the major IFs and the other focused on the Council of Europe. No permanent secretariat or organised focus. Limited organisational capacity and limited division of labour due to mutual suspicion.
An arena for the exchange of information, debate and regime maintenance.	Some regular forums, e.g. the Council of Europe Anti-doping Convention Monitoring Group and the IOC Medical Commission, but membership tended to be limited to either state or sport actors.

The establishment of WADA in the wake of the serious disruption to the 1998 Tour de France was a landmark in the development of a global anti-doping policy regime. Established in November 1999, WADA's mission is to:
"promote and co-ordinate at international level the fight against doping in sport in all its forms.... The Agency's principal task will be to co-ordinate a comprehensive anti-doping programme at international level, laying down common, effective, minimum standards, compatible with those in internationally recognised quality standards for doping controls...." (WADA 1999).

The establishment of WADA has done much to remedy the deficiencies in the policy regime identified in Table 1. WADA, with its representation from the major public and sports interests, and the formation of International Intergovernmental Consultative Group on Anti-Doping in Sport to co-ordinate the resources and views of public authorities, has given the regime greater stability and an enhanced capacity to fulfil the necessary functions for effective regime maintenance. WADA's potential has been partially realised by its prominent role in providing teams of observers to monitor and report on the effectiveness of doping control at major sports competitions. However, by far the most severe test of its potential to accomplish a quantum change in the success of anti-doping efforts is the successful implementation of the World Anti-Doping Code, a draft of which was published in June 2002, and consequently make progress towards the goal of harmonisation which is so evidently central to the Agency's mission. The purpose of this paper is to provide a brief overview of the draft Code and to reflect, in more detail, on the challenges that the pursuit of closer harmonisation will present.

The eight articles of the draft Code provide a mix of statements of values, principles, and procedural regulations designed to establish the Code as "the fundamental and universal document upon which the World Anti-Doping Program is based" (WADA 2002, para. 3.2). Article 5 is devoted to the comprehensive identification of stakeholders including athletes, their support personnel, governments, national Olympic committees, the IOC, the international federations, and event organising bodies. The Code specifies the primary roles and responsibilities of each group of stakeholders and identifies key areas for harmonisation including the definition of doping, international standards, covering technical and procedural aspects of doping control and laboratory analysis, principles governing hearings and appeals, determining when a violation of the anti-doping rules has occurred, and sanctions for doping violations. Each of these aspects of the Code is specified in varying degrees of detail and each raises particular issues in relation to the concept of harmonisation.

Over the last ten years or so a number of factors have combined to make closer harmonisation an imperative for successful anti-doping policy. First, there is a series of examples of athletes challenging a positive drug test on the grounds of inconsistency between the anti-doping rules of their home federation and those of the testing agency in the country in which they are training or competing (Houlihan 2002). Second, there is evidence of a large number of international federations that have poorly drafted and out-of-date anti-doping rules (Vrijman 1995; Siekmann et al. 1999). Third, the existence of overlapping jurisdictions has led to the inefficient use of scarce resources. Fourth, the need to reconcile two guiding principles, the first, usually adopted by state anti-doping agencies, is that athletes should be treated equally irrespective of their sport; and the second, generally adopted by international federations, means that athletes in each sport should be treated equally irrespective of nationality. Finally, there is the fact that legal challenge to the decision to impose sanctions is now routine rather than exceptional. The combined effect of these factors was to create suspicion and disillusion among athletes, irritation and frustration among governments, excessive caution and a preference for inaction among national sports federations, and confusion and cynicism among sports fans and the general public.

Unpacking harmonisation

Harmonisation is both an outcome and a process.[1] As an outcome harmonisation has a variety of possible meanings including technical uniformity, proximity, compatibility, and value consensus; as a process harmonisation might include collective negotiation, consultation and external imposition. Unfortunately, as an outcome harmonisation is a very vague concept. It is by no means easy to agree on the criteria by which harmonisation would be considered to have been achieved. Not only is there disagreement over the weight to be given to the different criteria, but the dynamic nature of doping in sport requires regular reassessment of the appropriateness of the policy mix. One purpose of publishing the World Anti-Doping Code is to set clear and public criteria for assessing harmonisation. Achieving the desired extent of harmonisation will require varying degrees of change in current policies and practices by stakeholders. One way of assessing the scale of the challenge facing WADA is to examine harmonisation in relation to the concepts of depth, breadth and intensity.

Depth

Depth has three distinct dimensions, the first of which refers to the extent of change required in government policies or those of IFs, for example in laws, regulations, administrative routines and the allocation of resources. To an extent many partners will seek to minimise the extent of change by adopting a "first mover" strategy (Héritier 1996), hoping that by taking the initiative in policy making they will be able to shape policy in such a way as to produce a "national [or organisational] home run" (Dimitrakopoulos & Richardson 2001: 344) which keeps the organisation's adjustment costs low. The IOC attempted this pre-emptive move at the Lausanne anti-doping conference in February 1999 when it suggested a global anti-doping agency under its control, but was forced to retreat due to pressure from a number of governments and the European Union.

With regard to this dimension of depth the challenges facing WADA in relation to some aspects of the Code are formidable. For example, in relation to the extent to which domestic legal systems are supportive of, or complementary to, the Code there is substantial variation, even among the members of the European Union where one might expect a greater degree of harmonisation of law regarding doping. There is variation with regard to access to drugs (in some countries access to drugs such as steroids are subject to tight legal control, by a Medicines Act, but in many countries access is only weakly controlled), possession of banned substances (some countries outlaw possession, but most do not), supply of banned substances (most countries outlaw supplying) and use of drugs in sport (only Italy has legislation to outlaw doping in sport). Countries generally display strong attachment to their pattern of domestic law, thus making change notoriously difficult. The Code stipulates that "Anti-doping rules should not be subject

BARRIE HOULIHAN

to, or limited by, the requirements and legal standards applicable to criminal proceedings or employment matters" (WADA 2002, para. 8.9.1). However, the drafters of the Code acknowledge the problem of asserting the superior status of the Code in relation to domestic law by the entreaty that: "The policies and minimum standards set forth in the Code represent the consensus of a broad spectrum of stakeholders with an interest in fair sport and should be respected by all courts and adjudicating bodies" (WADA 2002, para. 8.9.1).

Despite the degree of variation in funding, administrative arrangements and legal framework, the obstacles to achieving a greater depth of harmonisation should not be exaggerated. While there are marked global differences in administrative traditions, and especially between the more interventionist centralised state models, exemplified by France and Italy, the more interventionist decentralised state model as found in China regarding sport, and the more laissez faire model of countries such as the United States and the UK, there has been a gradual increase in the involvement of most states particularly with regard to the funding of anti-doping efforts, but also in securing more effective administrative arrangements. Examples include the establishment of anti-doping agencies in Canada and Australia and, most recently, the formation of the US Anti-Doping Agency. However, only about twenty-two countries have established publicly funded anti-doping agencies.

Similar variation exists between the major IFs with some, such as the IAAF and UCI, having a long history of leadership and innovation in doping control, though in the case of the UCI with a marked lack of success, and others, such as the ITF and FIFA, being far less enthusiastic. Although there has been some convergence of practice, there remains considerable variation in doping rules and procedures (Vrijman 1995; Siekmann et al 1999) and more profound variation in the intensity of commitment to pursue drug abusers. Finally, and perhaps most importantly, there is a growing divergence in the capacity of IFs to monitor and control the activities of domestic leagues, clubs and individual athletes. While some IFs retain considerable authority, others, particularly those responsible for the more commercial sports, such as football, rugby union, tennis, golf and road cycling, are seeing their authority steadily undermined.

The second dimension of depth concerns the degree to which international organisations such as the IOC and the international federations, but also governments, will have to adopt policies that they would not otherwise have adopted. The importance of this dimension goes to the heart of any discussion of harmonisation as it concerns the cost of compliance. Clearly harmonisation is easy to achieve if policy is specified in general terms and if thresholds are generous. The example of sanctions illustrates the nature of the problem, but also indicates the extent of convergence that has already taken place. As regards the severity of sanctions, there has been a long debate among the major federations and within the IOC about the appropriate sanctions for particular doping violations. For many years the norm in a number of key federations was four years for a first violation concerning steroids and a life ban for a subsequent violation. Recently the IOC recommended that the norm be reduced to two years for a first violation. One interpretation of the decision to halve the length of the ban was that it was an example of the attempt to achieve harmonisation by seeking the lowest common denominator, where policy is set at a point where even the least committed can comply with minimal change in their current policies. The view of the IOC was that a two- year ban was less likely to be challenged in domestic courts and therefore enabled consistency to be maintained. It was also argued by some doping control officials that the prospect of having to impose a four year ban made anti-doping authorities overly generous in giving athletes the benefit of the doubt. A further criticism of the imposition of a standard set of penalties for doping was that it failed to take account of the wide variation in the elite careers in different sports. An elite gymnast or figure skater may only have one or two opportunities to participate in an Olympic Games whereas a rower, middle distance runner or javelin thrower may compete in four or five Olympics. To impose a two year ban on a gymnast may represent the loss of 40% of his/her elite career, but only 10-15% of that of a javelin thrower.

The Code deals with sanctions by means of a sophisticated, and challenging compromise. Although the Code confirms a two-year disqualification as the minimum for a first violation, it allows for variation on grounds such as susceptibility to inadvertent use of some commonly available substances, therapeutic use, and lack of fault, thus addressing a number of concerns voiced by athletes in particular. However, periods of disqualification of less than two years are possible only on a case by case basis and with the onus clearly on the athlete to establish "that the doping violation was not the result of his or her fault or negligence" (WADA 2002, para. 8.8.3.2); and third parties to the Code would have discretion to impose additional sanctions "which are appropriate to the circumstances of the violation and the nature of the sport" (WADA 2002, para. 8.8.9). It is important to note that while the "nature of the sport" may be a basis for an increased sanction it is not allowable as a basis for a reduced sanction. This is an improvement on the IOC Anti-Doping Code which included the vague clause that allowed modification of the two year minimum suspension "based on specific, exceptional circumstances to be evaluated in the first instance by the competent IF bodies" (IOC 2000: 7).

The Code is thus an important attempt to achieve a balance in two important areas of policy. First, it is seeking to achieve balance between parity of treatment of athletes on the one hand and a recognition of the need for some capacity to vary sanctions due to the particular circumstances of the violation. Examples of grounds for variation might include where the athlete is very young or has taken a substance on the faulty advice of a doctor. The second area of balance is the attempt to retain some discretion and flexibility regarding sanctions while not creating the opportunity for an international federation, such as FIFA, to claim that its sport is an exception. While it is likely that the major Olympic IFs and activist governments will find the draft Code on sanctions acceptable in balancing minimum standards with discretion one or two major federations, FIFA in particular, are still likely to refuse the compromise.

Even assuming that there is acceptance of the two-year minimum ban and a common interpretation of the grounds for variation, there still remain many other aspects of the doping control process where negotiation over the depth of change in current practice will be required including, for example, the number of athletes selected for testing in particular sports, the frequency of testing, and how eligibility for testing is determined. In Britain, for example, while over 600 tests were conducted in 2001-02 in athletics, which has approximately 250 elite competitors, only 1016 tests were conducted in soccer, which has approximately 5000 elite players in England alone. Furthermore, approximately half the tests in soccer were for recreational drugs such as cocaine and marijuana and the tests were spread over the Premier League, the Nationwide League and youth and women's football rather than being concentrated at Premier League level. Given that there are about 500 footballers in the Premiership, the chances of a player competing at the highest level being tested for performance-enhancing drugs once in a season is remote. Even with the promise from the Football Association of 200 more tests in the 2001/02 season, the scale of testing does little to demonstrate the governing body's commitment to drug-free soccer.

The third dimension of depth is the extent to which the specification of policy prescription extends beyond general statements of values and addresses matters of operational detail. In a policy area as complex and dynamic as doping, with multiple stakeholders and a need to cope with exceptional cases, it is likely that there will be some elements that require specification at the level of values or principles, but there will also be elements that will require much more detailed specification. I have suggested elsewhere (Houlihan 1999a) that there are four distinct levels or interpretations of harmonisation namely, as uniformity, proximity, compatibility and consensus (see Table 2), though in the light of the content of the Code it is necessary to add a fifth, namely tolerability.

Table 2: Varieties of harmonisation.

Intended outcome	Description	Examples from the World Anti-Doping Code
Uniformity	Identical standards or processes	Art. 2: definition of doping Art. 3.3: the use of International Standards for "technical and operational parts of the anti-doping program"
Proximity	Very close similarity in standards and processes, with variation justified by the particularities of countries, sports or events.	Art 5.3.7: requires the regulation of import, export, manufacture and labelling of prohibited substances, but leaves the precise form of regulation to individual governments. Art 5.12.5: the conduct of hearings arising from an alleged doping violation shall be in accord with the rules of the anti-doping agency initiating the urine test

Compatibility	Difference is allowed up to the point where it undermines the credibility of standards, processes and objectives and breaches agreed basic principles.	Art 3.4: models of best practice will be "recommended by WADA but they will not be mandatory for parties accepting the Code" Art 8.3.5: parties to the Code may test for additional substances Art 8.8.9: "Parties accepting the Code may, at their discretion, choose to adopt rules imposing additional sanctions for anti-doping rule violations"
Consensus	Agreement on values and ends, which allows for a variation in means.	Art 1: which list a set of fundamental values for sport
Tolerability	Acceptable disharmony	Art. 4.3.3: non-compliance is tolerated "if the explanation is justified by lack of financial resources, supervening law which the party has no power to change, or other justification acceptable to WADA"

Table 2 shows that the drafters of the Code have used the full range of interpretations of harmonisation. As is only to be expected, the strictest interpretation, uniformity, is reserved for those aspects where legal challenge is likely and where scientific precision is important. The use of standards approved by the International Standards Organisation is common among European businesses and was a central element of the International Anti-Doping Arrangement, but is far less common in the United States where externally developed standards are more likely to be perceived as unwelcome regulation. In a number of important areas the Code relies on proximity, especially where anti-doping agencies have well established procedures and protocols. In some areas, such as the conduct of hearings, the Code does specify a reasonably precise set of expectations and well recognised principles to guide action. However, in other areas, such as the role of the government in controlling access to drugs and supplements, the Code is more vague in that it uses words such as "regulation," which are open to wide interpretation.

Harmonisation as compatibility is also widely adopted within the Code, though it is mainly used to enable variation from recommended or required practices if the intention is to give added rigour. For example, sanctions above the minimum specified in the Code may be imposed by the parent International Federation for particular classes of violation. Harmonisation as consensus is most evident in Article One which seeks to capture the "spirit of sport" through the listing of a series of statements, some more persuasive than others. Sport is claimed variously to be the builder of communities, a pathway to health, and a source of international peace. Although many of the assertions are based, at best, on contradictory empirical evidence, they are only plausible as a set of laudable aspirations. There is a final interpretation, that of tolerability, that stretches the definition of harmonisation to its limit and refers to those elements of the Code where a level of disharmony is acceptable. Given that so much of the Code is, and clearly has to be, tightly prescriptive, there is always the danger that full implementation and compliance will prove extremely difficult for many stakeholders. The drafters of the Code were wise, therefore, to build in some flexibility in determining compliance. It is likely that the definition of what "justification [for non-compliance] is acceptable to WADA" (Art. 4.3.3) will take some time to be refined through "case law."

Breadth

Breadth refers to the proportion of potential parties to an agreement that is deemed sufficient for satisfactory implementation. Few would argue that full compliance of all 199 countries that participated in the Sydney Games is necessary for the implementation of the World Anti-Doping Code. Most would also agree that the success of the Code is not even dependent on acceptance by all eighty medal-winning countries at Sydney or the twenty-five at Salt Lake City. Indeed, it is possible to argue that the success of the Code is dependent upon a relatively small number of countries. As Table 3 shows, the number of countries that win more than one or two medals is small. Although eighty countries won at least one medal at the 2000 Games, only thirty-two countries accounted for 90% of the medals total. Similarly, at the 2002 Winter Games, ten countries, which were also in the most successful thirty-two at the summer Games, won almost 75% of all medals. It can therefore be argued that implementation relies on the acceptance of the Code by only thirty or so major "sports powers."

Table 3: Distribution of medals at the 2000 Olympic Games and 2002 Winter Games.

At Sydney 2000, of the 80 medal-winning countries:
  16 (20%) won 72.5% of the medals
  32 (40%) won 90% of the medals

At Sydney 2000, of the 199 participating countries:
  40 (20%) won 94.7% of the medals

At Salt Lake City 2002, of the 25 medal-winning countries:
  10 (40%) won 74.8% of the medals

At Salt Lake City 2002, of the 77 participating countries:
  23 (30%) won 99.2% of the medals

Breadth can also refer to the scope or pervasiveness of the policy. If Olympic sports constitute the core focus for anti-doping policy, how far beyond that core should the policy extend? Not surprisingly, WADA is giving priority to Olympic sports and Olympic-level competition, but assuming successful implementation of the Code by 2004 it is inevitable that WADA will begin to discuss the extent of its responsibility for doping beyond the Olympic movement. This is clearly the direction that the EU would like to see WADA move, and it would also be consistent with the WADA mission statement.

Intensity

The third dimension, intensity, refers to the level of commitment of key organisations and governments. Both sports organisations and governments have a wide range of responsibilities and demands on their resources. Inevitably, the issue of doping may not remain as their primary concern over the long term. If it is accepted that the intensity of interest and commitment of time and other resources will vary, the acceptable limits of that variation need to be specified. In other words, what is the maximum acceptable level of under-compliance? More importantly, the strategy for implementation of the Code needs to address directly the question of maintaining policy commitment. At present, governments are considering their responses to the draft Code, and a number of governments which have traditionally been in the forefront of anti-doping efforts, such as Norway and Switzerland, are voicing serious reservations about their ability to accept the Code in its entirety, largely because of the specific nature of many of the obligations that they would have to undertake.

Conclusion

The long-standing difficulty in agreeing on an acceptable and legally robust list of sanctions is indicative of the general problems facing WADA in drafting the Code and in achieving its acceptance. As with the list of sanctions, the search is not for an ideal Code but for an optimal document which balances the competing interests of the various stakeholders and which acknowledges the reality of domestic and international sports politics. In many respects, the drafters of the Code have demonstrated considerable subtlety in using the full range of interpretations of harmonisation in the preparation of the Code. Evaluated within the immediate context of the 1999 Lausanne anti-doping conference from which the idea of WADA emerged, the Code achieves a fine balance between the twin imperatives of seeking the most rigorous and robust standards in doping control and in gaining the acceptance of the Code by the vast majority of the Olympic sports federations and the thirty-five or so main "sports powers."

However, as with much policy-making, there is often a narrow window of opportunity for success when the variety of factors in the policy environment are at their most auspicious. The particular co-incidence in 1999 of defensiveness on the part of the IOC and the international federations, and a high level of governmental interest in doping, particularly from the United States and the EU, created uniquely favourable conditions for the strengthening of the global anti-doping regime. The co-incidence of factors conducive to change was sufficient to overcome first, the deeply entrenched inertia among key actors such as the national Olympic committees, which have rarely, if ever, taken a lead in anti-doping efforts; second, the equivocation of the IOC; and third, the ambivalence of many governments which, on the one hand, want to protect the utility of international sporting competition as a viable political and economic resource and, on the other hand, want to ensure that they have a sufficient number of successful elite athletes to be in a position to exploit that resource.

The key concern for supporters of drug-free sport is whether the momentum that developed in the wake of the 1998 Tour de France doping scandal can be sustained to ensure acceptance and effective implementation of the Code. While WADA has rapidly established itself as a respected and assertive organisation, there are some signs that the policy context is not quite as propitious as it once was, as some key policy actors are less enthusiastic than they were in 1999. The election of centre-right governments in Italy, France and the United States has led to a distinct loss of governmental commitment to anti-doping efforts, partly due to the general suspicion of regulation and state intervention that characterise contemporary centre-right parties, but also to the growing evidence that the issue is simply less salient than four years ago. The current French minister responsible for sport, Jean-Francois Lamour, has spoken critically of the high priority that his predecessor, Marie-George Buffet, gave to the issue of doping, George Bush has shown less interest in the issue of doping in sport than did Bill Clinton, and Silvio Berlusconi has done little to strengthen the anti-doping work of CONI. Another key actor, the IOC, appears content to watch the activities of WADA from the sidelines as though it were not an integral part of the Agency. Even the EU's relationship with WADA has gone through a difficult period due to disagreements over funding. Unless the key sports powers in North America and Europe, the IOC and the major IFs are far more explicit in their support for the Code, it is likely that the current target dates for acceptance will prove significantly over-ambitious. The fate of the Code rests not just on the skill of the drafting committee, which has been considerable, but also on the political will and leadership of a small number of key governments, many of which were the same governments that were so quick to condemn the IOC for its lack of leadership on doping at the 1999 Lausanne conference.

References

Dimitrakopoulos, D. & Richardson, J. (2001) Implementing EU public policy. In European Union: Power and policy-making (ed.) J. Richardson, London: Routledge.

International Olympic Committee (2000) Anti-Doping Code, Lausanne: IOC.

Héritier, A. (1996) The accommodation of diversity in European policy-making and its outcomes: Regulatory policy as patchwork, Journal of European Public Policy, 3.2, pp.149-67.

Houlihan, B. (1999) Dying to Win: Doping in sport and the development of anti-doping policy, Strasbourg: Council of Europe Publishing.

Houlihan, B. (1999a) Policy harmonisation: The example of global anti-doping policy, Journal of Sport Management, 13, pp 197-215.

Houlihan, B. (2002) (2nd edition) Dying to Win: Doping in sport and the development of anti-doping policy, Strasbourg: Council of Europe Publishing.

Krasner, S. (1983) Structural causes and regime consequences: Regimes as intervening variables. In S. Krasner (ed.) International regimes, pp. 1-21, Ithaca, NY: Cornell University Press.

Siekmann, R.R.C, Soek, J. & Bellani, A. (1999) (eds.) Doping rules of international sports organisations, The Hague: TMC Asser/Kluwer.

Vrijman, E.N. (1995) Harmonisation: Can it Ever Really be Achieved?, Strasbourg: Council of Europe, 1995.

WADA (1999) Mission statement, Lausanne, WADA.

WADA (2002) Draft outline for the World Anti-doping Code, E-version 1.0, Montreal: WADA.

Notes

1 For a fuller discussion of the problems of policy harmonisation in doping see Houlihan, B. (1999).

CHAPTER 2

DOPING IN SPORT: SOME ISSUES FOR MEDICAL PRACTITIONERS

Ivan Waddington

It is generally agreed that the era of modern doping in sport dates from the 1950s and 1960s. It is also clear that, since then, the use of performance-enhancing substances in sport has become increasingly common. The central objects of this paper are (i) to examine some aspects of this increase in the use of performance-enhancing drugs and, more particularly, to analyse the role of sports physicians in that process and (ii) to examine the limitations of current anti-doping policies, some of the alternatives to current policies and the implications of these alternative policies for doctors.

The growing competitiveness of modern sport

One of the key social processes associated with the increase in the use of performance-enhancing drugs in sport since the Second World War has been the growing competitiveness of modern sport. This process, in turn, has been associated with a number of broader social processes, of which the politicisation of sport and the massive increases in the rewards – particularly the financial rewards – associated with sporting success have been of particular significance. Both these processes have had the consequence of increasing the competitiveness of sport, one aspect of which has involved the downgrading, in relative terms, of the traditional value associated with taking part whilst greatly increasing the value attached to winning.

The medicalisation of sport

A second key process associated with the increasing use of performance-enhancing drugs in sport has been the growing involvement of physicians in the medical management of athletes. This process has been described as the medicalisation of sport (Waddington, 2000) and is an aspect of the medicalisation of society more generally.

It is primarily on this process of the medicalisation of sport that I wish to focus in this paper.

The medicalisation process in society more generally has involved growing dependence on professionally provided care and on drugs, the medicalisation of prevention and the medicalisation of the expectations of lay people regarding health-related issues. In recent years, the medicalisation process has enveloped sport. Central to the medicalisation of sport has been the development, particularly since the 1960s, of sports medicine, which is premised on the idea that highly trained athletes have special medical needs and therefore require special medical supervision.

As Houlihan (1999) has noted, the development of sports medicine has been associated with the development of a culture which encourages the treatment not just of injured athletes, but also of healthy athletes, with drugs. He notes that:

> Even if the 'drugs' are simply those which are legally available (in terms defined by both the state and the IOC), such as vitamins and food supplements, the athlete is already developing the expectations and patterns of behaviour that might initially parallel illegal drug use, but which are to most athletes part of a common culture (Houlihan, 1999:88).

This point was nicely illustrated by Robert Voy, former chief medical officer for the US Olympic Committee, when he recorded the daily intake of legal drugs of a national track star: vitamin E, 160mg; B-complex capsules, four times per day; vitamin C, 2000 mg; vitamin B6, 150 mg; calcium tablets, four times per day; magnesium tablets, twice a day; zinc tablets, three times a day; royal jelly capsules; garlic tablets; cayenne tablets; eight aminos; Gamma-Oryzanol; Mega Vit Pack; super-charge herbs; Dibencozide; glandular tissue complex; natural steroid complex; Inosine; Orchid testicle extract; Pyridium; Ampicillin; and hair rejuvenation formula with Biotin (Voy, 1991:99).

It is important to emphasise that the relationship between athletes and sports medicine practitioners goes beyond the treatment of sports injuries for, as the British Medical Association's (1996:4) definition of sports medicine indicates, sports medicine is concerned not just with the 'prevention, diagnosis, and treatment of exercise related illnesses and injuries' but also with the 'maximization of performance'. Moreover, as the rewards associated with winning have increased, so the role of sports medicine practitioners in maximizing performance has also become more important. One consequence of this growing concern of sports physicians with the maximization of performance (Hoberman, 1992) has been to make top-class athletes more and more dependent on increasingly sophisticated systems of medical support in their efforts to run faster, to jump further or higher or to compete more effectively in their chosen sport; indeed, as the head of the IOC Medical Commission observed in 1976, "Modern top competition is unimaginable without doctors" (cited in Todd and Todd, 2000:74) and, at the highest levels, the quality of medical support may make the difference between success and failure. Brown and Benner for example, have pointed out that, as increased importance has been placed on winning, so athletes:

have turned to mechanical (exercise, massage), nutritional (vitamins, minerals), psycho-logical (discipline, transcendental meditation), and pharmacological (medicines, drugs) methods to increase their advantage over opponents in competition. A major emphasis has been placed on the nonmedical use of drugs, particularly anabolic steroids, central nervous system stimulants, depressants and analgesics. (Brown and Benner, 1984:32).

The sport-medicine axis

Sports medicine is a legitimate area of specialist practice. There is, however, a substantial and well documented history of the involvement of sports physicians in the development and use of performance-enhancing drugs. Prominent – indeed, infamous – examples of medical involvement include the central role of Dr John Ziegler, the US team doc-tor at the 1954 World Games in Vienna, in the development and dissemination among the weightlifting community of the first widely used anabolic steroids; the systematic involvement of doctors in doping in the former East Germany; and the involvement of sports medicine specialists in the development of blood doping (Waddington, 2000).

As long ago as 1988, a leading UK medical journal, the *Lancet,* published an article under the title *Sports medicine – is there lack of control?* It suggested that although "evidence of direct involvement of medical practitioners in the procurement and ad-ministration of hormones is lacking, their connivance with those who do so is obvious and their participation in blood doping is a matter of record." It concluded:

> Members of the medical profession have long been concerned with the health and welfare of people in sport, but never have the stakes been so high. Evidence continues to grow that some are showing more interest in finding new ways of enhancing the performance of those in their charge than in their physical wellbeing (1988: 612).

Two years after that *Lancet* editorial, the Dubin Commission of Inquiry in Canada docu-mented the involvement of substantial numbers of sports physicians in providing per-formance-enhancing drugs to athletes in many sports and in several countries. The Com-mission found that, in Canada, the "names of physicians willing to prescribe anabolic steroids and other performance-enhancing drugs circulate widely in gyms" and that "there are physicians in most major centres across the country who have at one time or another been involved in prescribing anabolic steroids and other performance-enhancing drugs to athletes" (Dubin, 1990:357). It noted that the situation in the United States was similar to that in Canada, while evidence provided to the Commission on the situation in Australia indicated that in that country drugs were also readily available from physicians.

If the Dubin Commission marked one watershed in the history of the use of per-formance-enhancing drugs, then the 1998 Tour de France may come to be regarded as a second watershed, particularly in terms of the amount of information that was made available about the systematic and organised use of performance-enhancing drugs in professional cycling and about the pivotal role of team doctors in this process (Waddington, 2000:153-169).

Perhaps not surprisingly, almost all the media coverage of the doping scandal in that Tour was heavily emotive and did little to enhance our understanding of the processes involved. One exception, which brought out particularly clearly the involvement of team doctors, was a piece written for *The Times* by James Waddington, a novelist who is also a cycling fan. Waddington pointed to the enormous physical demands which the Tour makes upon riders and suggested that, in the attempt to keep their team members in the race, team doctors will draw upon an exhaustive knowledge of a range of substances – nutritional, hormonal and anabolic. He continued:

> It is a complex regime, with maybe 20 different components ... Only the team doctor has this exhaustive knowledge, and thus the average professional cyclist with no scientific background becomes not a partner but a patient. He opens his mouth, holds out his arm, and trusts. That trust, not the reflex shriek of 'drugs, the excrement of Satan', should be the crucial point in the whole discussion (*Times*, 25 July, 1998).

One might take issue with Waddington's characterisation of professional cyclists as passive participants in this process, but he does make a point which is of fundamental importance: *if we wish to understand the use of performance-enhancing drugs in sport then it is crucial that we understand the centrality of the relationship between elite level athletes and practitioners of sports medicine.*

This point was clearly brought out by Cramer in his report on the use of blood doping by the United States cycling team at the 1984 Olympics. After the Olympics it was revealed that most of the American team, which had dominated the cycling events, had been blood doped and, shortly afterwards, the technique was banned by the International Olympic Committee (IOC). Cramer wrote:

> In the national euphoria after the games, no one thought to pry out any secrets. The US team had won nine medals, dominating the cycling events. 'Great riders ...' 'Great coach ...' 'Great bikes ...' said the press, reporting the daisy chain of back pats. No one thought to add, 'Great doctors ...'. (Cramer, 1985:25)

The regulation of doping

The first compulsory Olympic drug testing took place at the 1968 Winter Games, and since then anti-doping policies in sport have been based on what might be described as a "law and order" approach, in which emphasis has been placed on the detection and punishment of offenders.

How successful have such policies been? This question is not easy to answer, not least because the objectives of anti-doping policies are rarely clearly defined. However, the following points should be noted in any attempt to evaluate the effectiveness of such policies.

Firstly, Voy (1991) has drawn attention to what he calls a "sad paradox" of anti-doping policies. He notes that the severe punishments which often follow detection of drug use constrain drug-using athletes to place primary importance on the detectability of drugs rather than on their safety; as a consequence, anti-doping controls have pushed athletes towards the use of drugs which may be more dangerous, but less detectable) It is probably fair to conclude that this was not the intention of those who devised these controls.

Secondly, it has been argued (Black, 1996) that the ban on the use of performance-enhancing drugs makes it difficult for users to obtain medical advice and monitoring in relation to their use of drugs. This consideration may not apply to drug-using elite athletes who work in cooperation with team physicians, but it is certainly the case that at the non-elite level there is an unmet medical need on the part of drug users for qualified, confidential and non-judgemental medical advice (Korkia and Stimson, 1993). I will return to this issue later.

Thirdly, there is no evidence to suggest that the ban on doping has effectively controlled the use of performance-enhancing drugs) It is of course difficult to arrive at a precise estimate of the prevalence of doping. However, the available evidence suggests by the mid-1970s, performance-enhancing drugs had already come to be regarded as an essential aid to training and/or competition by many athletes (Coni *et al.*, 1988:Para. B14) and that, since then, their use has become even more widespread.

In her evidence presented to the US Senate Judiciary Committee Hearing on Steroid Abuse in America, Pat Connolly, a coach of the US women's track and field team, estimated that of the fifty members of the team at the 1984 Olympics, "probably 15 of them had used steroids. Some of them were medalists." Asked whether the number of athletes using steroids had increased by the time of the Seoul Olympics of 1988, Connolly replied "Oh, yes. Oh, yes, it went up a lot." She estimated that: "At least 40 per cent of the women's team in Seoul had probably used steroids at some time in their preparation for the games" (cited in Dubin, 1990: 339).

Shortly before this US Senate Judiciary Committee hearing, the Australian government, concerned about the apparently increasing use of banned substances by athletes, referred the issue to a Senate standing committee for investigation and report. The committee heard evidence that approximately 70% of Australian athletes who competed internationally had taken drugs and that one quarter of the Australian track and field team at the Seoul Olympics had used drugs (Australian Parliament, 1989:75).

The most systematic and reliable evidence on the extent of doping in elite sport is that which was presented to the Dubin Commission of Inquiry in Canada. Dubin concluded:

After hearing evidence and meeting with knowledgeable people from Canada, the United States, Australia, New Zealand, and elsewhere, I am convinced that the problem is widespread not only in Canada but also around the world. The evidence shows that banned performance-enhancing substances and, in particular, anabolic steroids are being used by athletes in almost every sport, most extensively in weightlifting and track and field (Dubin, 1990: 336).

There is no evidence to suggest that the problem has lessened in the last few years. Anthony Millar, Research Director at the Institute of Sports Medicine in Sydney, Australia, wrote in 1996 of an "epidemic of drug usage" in sport, and suggested that the use of performance-enhancing drugs 'is widespread and growing not only in the athletic community but also among recreational athletes' (Millar, 1996:107-108). In a survey of 448 British Olympic athletes, carried out in 1995, 48 percent felt that drug use was a problem in international competition in their sport (in track and field, the figure was 86 percent). Nor did these elite British athletes feel that the problem was being effectively tackled by the existing system of doping controls; 23 per cent of athletes felt drug use had increased over the previous twelve months compared to just 6 per cent who felt it had decreased (Sports Council, 1996:34). More recently, the revelations about doping in the 1998 Tour de France provided unambiguous evidence that doping in professional cycling is both widespread and systematically organized (Waddington, 2000:153-69). It is also clear that drugs are widely used in other sport-related contexts. In a British survey of anabolic steroid use in 'hardcore' gyms (defined as gyms having predominantly heavy weight training equipment, competitive bodybuilders and relatively few female members), over 29% of gym users were currently using anabolic steroids (Lenehan *et al.*, 1996). Charles Walker, Head of Sports in the Council of Europe, has estimated that in a city the size of London "there will be at least 30,000 and probably as many as 60,000 regular users of anabolic steroids" (Walker, 1994).

Towards a new anti-doping policy?

The review of evidence outlined above suggests that doping is widespread in many sports and that in some sports it is very widespread. If it can be assumed that a central objective of anti-doping policies is to control the use by athletes of performance-enhancing drugs, then it would seem reasonable to conclude that current anti-doping policy has not worked well. This is not to suggest that current anti-doping controls should be dismantled and that athletes should be allowed to take any substances without regulation; apart from health-related objections to such a policy, an extremely liberal policy of this kind is simply not politically realistic and would be likely to produce a flight from sport by both public and private sponsors who would not wish to be associated with an activity in which the open use of drugs was accepted. However, there are a number of other policy options which might be explored. One of these involves a movement towards harm reduction policies. As Coomber (1996) has noted, many of the public health issues involved in the use of drugs in sport are not dissimilar to those involved in the use of drugs in a non-sporting context. Thus athletes "may be using unsafe ways of administering their drugs, using unsafe drugs in unsafe ways, and may even be unintentional transmission routes into the non-sporting world of sexually transmitted diseases such as HIV" (Coomber,1996:18). Outside of the sporting context, public health authorities in many countries have sought to deal with problems of this kind by the development of *harm reduction* policies. Coomber describes the development of these policies in Britain as follows:

> With the advent of HIV/AIDS in the non-sporting world, drug policy … concerned itself with reducing the spread of HIV to the general population. This meant accessing one of the high-risk groups likely to spread the virus – injecting drug users – who had contracted high levels of infection due to needle-sharing practices. Access to this group, and introducing them to practices likely to reduce the spread of the virus … took priority over compelling these people to stop using drugs. Without access to non-judgemental help and real benefits (such as clean needles, and in some circumstances even access to drugs of choice), these users, who were not interested in stopping using drugs, would not have been accessed. A major policy decision was made that HIV represented a bigger threat to Public Health than drug use" (Coomber, 1996:19).

Harm reduction includes a variety of strategies, with needle exchange schemes as a central aspect of such policies. Rather than attempting to *eliminate* drug use – an unrealistic target – the goal is to reduce harm. Harm reduction policies are already well established in a number of countries, including the Netherlands, Switzerland and Britain (Goode, 1997:81) and there is growing interest in harm reduction schemes throughout Europe and beyond. The Thirteenth International Conference on the Reduction of Drug-related Harm was held in Ljubljana, Slovenia, in March 2002, while international guidelines for health protection in nightclubs were adopted at the Second International Conference on Nightlife Substance Abuse and Related Health Issues, held in Rimini, Italy, in March 2002. The meeting adopted the Rimini Declaration, which set out a series of safe-clubbing guidelines aimed at minimising the most frequent drug-related health hazards to young club-goers (EMCDDA, 2002). The European Monitoring Centre for Drugs and Drug Addiction (EMCDDA) also recently reported a trend in drug legislation in member states of the European Union, involving a shift away from traditional repressive policies and towards an emphasis on providing assistance and treatment for addicts (EMCDDA, 2002). Some aspects of policy in the United States (for example, the methadone replacement programmes for heroin addicts) might also be considered as a move away from traditional punitive policies.

However, within the sporting world, anti-drugs policy has been almost exclusively of the punitive, 'law and order' kind, and little thought has been given to the development of harm reduction policies. Coomber suggests that one reason for this is that those responsible for making and implementing anti-doping policy in sport "do not, in general, work within the same parameters as those policy makers outside sport … Drug policy in sport is seen as an issue that concerns sport and sporting authorities, and it has essentially isolated itself from considerations of how drug policy in sport relates to the world outside of it" (Coomber, 1996:17-18). He adds:

> There are many lessons to be learned about drugs, drug users and methods of control from the non-sporting world but those who make policy about drugs in sport are not drug policy experts, they are sport administrators. Those that are drug experts are often in fact literally just that; they are chemists and are often equally unaware of *broader* policy issues. This is patently obvious in the continued approach to sporting drug policy. It is bereft of ideas (because it is bereft of broader drug policy knowledge and experience), and it is putting people in danger by being so (Coomber, 1996:18).

What, then, would a harm reduction policy in sport look like, and what might be the advantages of such a policy? This question is not an entirely hypothetical one, for there have recently been some small but important movements in sport towards harm reduction policies. Let us begin by examining some recent developments in professional cycling.

That cycling is the first sport to move towards harm reduction policies is not perhaps surprising and can be explained largely in terms of two considerations. Firstly, as we noted earlier, doping is extremely common in professional cycling; indeed, it is possible that doping is more widespread in cycling than in any other sport. In this sense, the failure of traditional anti-doping policies is perhaps more clear in cycling than in any other sport. Secondly, not only is doping widespread, but one of the drugs most widely used – erythropoietin, commonly called EPO – carries very substantial health risks; indeed, EPO may well be the most dangerous, in health terms, of all the performance-enhancing drugs currently available.

EPO substantially boosts the performance of endurance athletes by stimulating the production of red blood cells. However, while EPO has a valuable medical use for patients with thin blood, its use in healthy people can produce a dangerous thickening of the blood which can result in blood clots leading to heart failure. EPO came onto the market in Europe in 1987 and it was followed almost immediately by a sudden spate of deaths from heart failure among professional cyclists. Between 1987 and 1990, fourteen Dutch riders and four Belgians – all young and apparently healthy elite athletes – died suddenly and the overwhelming probability is that most, if not all, of these unexpected deaths were associated with the use of EPO (*Independent on Sunday*, July 14, 1991); that all the deaths occurred amongst Dutch and Belgian riders also suggests the establishment of an early EPO 'grapevine' and distribution network in Holland and Belgium, though the use of EPO has since become commonplace among professional riders throughout Europe.

Concern about the widespread use of drugs within cycling and, probably more importantly, concern about the particular health threat posed by EPO, appears to have stimulated a rethink of anti-doping policy in cycling in much the same way that the particular health threat associated with HIV/AIDS stimulated the development of harm reduction policies in relation to drug control more generally. Hein Verbruggen, the President of the governing body of professional cycling, the Union Cycliste Internationale (UCI), announced in February 1997 a significant shift in policy, involving a move away from traditional anti-doping policy and towards a policy based on the principles of occupational health and harm reduction.

ᐟ(The system introduced by the UCI involves the taking of blood samples from riders shortly before major races. Blood tests then determine the level of haematocrit – the amount of red blood cells – in a rider's blood, and any rider with an haematocrit level which is considered to be dangerous to health – defined by the UCI as above 50% – is not allowed to start that race or any other race until a further test has indicated that the rider's haematocrit level has dropped to within safe limits)ᐟ

Verbruggen emphasised the non-punitive, harm reduction and occupational health aspects of the new policy:

> For us, the blood test is a health test. The UCI medical commission has been thinking about it for years but it has been impossible because you need blood tests, and they can't be imposed. What we have dreamed of is doing the same thing in cycling as is done in a normal working relationship between employer and employee. There are certain things the employer is obliged to take care of: for example, ear protection if you are working somewhere with a lot of noise …
>
> Where a guy works in a paint factory and is found to have too much lead in his blood, he is released from his job, and has to get better before he can come back. For years, we thought about making the teams responsible for the riders' health, as other employers are … We're in a tough sport and we should control the health of our riders (*Cycle Sport*, April 1997:30).

Verbruggen emphasised that the test was not an anti-doping test as such, but rather a health test. Noting that the effect which one gets with EPO can also be obtained by altitude training or by using an oxygen chamber, Verbruggen stated:

> You can have long, intellectual discussions about why you have to forbid EPO but accept riders training at altitude, which has exactly the same effect. The bad thing is the risk, the danger … You limit the risk by saying, "Wait a moment, we're not going to worry if it's EPO, an oxygen chamber or altitude training, if your haematocrit level is over 50, you don't start" (*Cycle Sport*, April 1997:30).

It might be noted that, unlike the first doping tests in cycling, which were introduced in the 1960s and which were met with riders' strikes, the new health tests were brought in with the agreement of the riders and teams, a fact which is almost certainly associated with the non-punitive character of the tests.

It might also be noted that some other organizations have recently adopted the policy of "health tests" pioneered by the Union Cycliste Internationale. Following the 1998 Tour de France, the French Cycling Federation not only adopted, but extended, the principle of health checks; all elite riders on French teams are now given an in-depth health check every three months to reveal and investigate physical changes. The results of the second of these health tests revealed that half of the riders in French teams (67 out of 135 on whom the tests were done) had been temporarily excluded from racing for a variety of reasons, principally abnormally high iron levels but also because of kidney problems and abnormal red blood cell counts. Speaking to *Le Monde*, the doctor to the French Federation, Armand Megret, stated that the results "would seem to indicate abuse of substances of all kinds, but not necessarily illegal ones, like, for example, the excessive intake of iron. This can be dangerous, even after stopping taking these products" (*Cycling Weekly*, 5 June, 1999).

A system of "health checks" has also recently been introduced by the Italian Olympic Committee (CONI) as part of a programme entitled *Io non rischio la salute* (I'm not risking my health). These health tests, involving analysis of blood and urine samples, have been carried out on various Italian sportspeople, including footballers, athletes, rowers and basketball players (*Cycling Weekly*, 29 May, 1999).

Another harm reduction scheme worthy of examination is that in operation in County Durham in the north of England. In January 1994, the County Durham Health Authority began funding a mobile needle exchange scheme which was targeted at inject-ing drug users and which was designed in the first instance as part of a harm reduction policy in relation to the transmission of HIV infection. To the surprise of the organ-izers of the needle exchange scheme, it quickly became clear that a majority of those using the scheme were bodybuilders who were using anabolic steroids. Some users of anabolic steroids had been attracted to the scheme because they had been unable to get medical help and advice from their regular physicians, some of whom had responded to requests for help in a hostile and heavily judgemental fashion and had refused to offer any advice until the bodybuilders stopped using steroids. With this evidence of unmet medical need, County Durham Health Authority established, in early 1995, a "drugs and sport" clinic.

The clinic now has approximately 450 clients, most of whom are bodybuilders. It provides a confidential and non-judgemental service to users of anabolic steroids and other performance-enhancing drugs, and the policy goals of the clinic centre around harm reduction rather than cessation of drug use. New clients are given an initial as-sessment in relation to their pattern of drug use and sexual health (the latter mainly in respect of HIV transmission) followed by a physical examination which includes blood sample analysis for a red blood cell count and a lipid profile. In addition, clients are monitored for liver function. Clients are encouraged to ensure that the intervals between cycles of drug use are such as to minimise the health risks and are also given advice, for example in relation to diet, which may help them to achieve their desired body shape with lower doses of drugs, or perhaps by using less dangerous drugs. A confidential counselling service is also provided for anabolic steroid users who experience side-effects such as sexual dysfunction or aggression (British Medical Association, 2002: 104). Broadly similar schemes are in operation in Wirral, Cheshire, and in Nottingham and Cardiff and an increasing number of agencies have workers in the field targeting anabolic steroid users (Korkia and Stimson, 1993:112-3).

What lessons can be learned from such schemes? Should sporting and/or public medical authorities consider the more widespread funding of such schemes as part of a harm reduction policy? What might be some of the consequences of a reorientation on the part of sporting bodies towards harm reduction policies? And what might be some of the objections to such a shift in policy?

At the outset it should be acknowledged that a reorientation of policy along these lines would not be unproblematic. However, if we are honest we should also recognise that the issue of drug use and control is, as Goode has pointed out, one where there may be no ideal solution and that it may well be that we are forced to accept "the least bad of an array of very bad options" (Goode, 1997:ix).

One possible objection to harm reduction policies is that such policies, it might be argued, imply condoning the use of drugs. In response to possible objections of this kind, it might be noted that such arguments were also voiced when harm reduction policies, such as needle exchange schemes, were initially developed in relation to drug control policies more generally. Although such arguments are still occasionally heard, the case for needle exchange schemes has now generally been accepted in Britain, and such schemes have been funded by governments – both Conservative and Labour – which no one could legitimately accuse of having adopted a "soft" or permissive policy in relation to drug use in general. Thus the shift towards harm reduction policies is not incompatible with, and does not imply the dismantling of, more conventional forms of drug control. In Britain, for example, the development of needle exchange schemes has not been accompanied by any relaxation of laws relating to the possession or sale of controlled drugs such as marijuana, heroin or cocaine.

What health benefits might be associated with harm reduction policies? One obvious benefit associated with "sport and drugs" clinics of the kind outlined above is that they provide what is clearly a much needed service to those using performance-enhancing drugs, whether in sport or other sport-related activities, not least in the fact that they provide qualified, confidential and non-judgemental medical advice which otherwise might be difficult to obtain. Though many drug-using athletes at the elite level undoubtedly receive qualified medical advice and monitoring it is clear that, below this level, there is a considerable unmet demand for medical support. A study carried out in British gyms indicated that users of anabolic steroids generally felt that most medical practitioners had little knowledge of their use and were unable to provide unbiased information on different drugs and their effects on health. The researchers found that "the majority of AS [anabolic steroid] users would welcome medical involvement but are unable to get the supervision they would like" (Korkia and Stimson, 1993:113).

Perhaps not surprisingly, medical practitioners were not an important source of advice for most users of anabolic steroids, the major sources of information being friends (35.8%), followed by anabolic steroid handbooks (25.7%) and dealers (20.2%). There are undoubtedly health risks associated with this pattern of obtaining information; Korkia and Stimson (1993:110-111) noted, for example, that steroid users would sometimes recommend doping practices different from those they used themselves (in order not to reveal their "secret for success") while some men may provide advice to women based on their – the men's – own experiences, which could have serious consequences for female anabolic steroid users in terms of virilising effects. Again, the provision of specialist medical advice on a confidential and non-judgemental basis might have considerable benefits in terms of harm reduction.

In a recent report, the British Medical Association (2002) suggested that harm reduction schemes of this kind merit further consideration by those concerned with the health of athletes. However, it is important to note that such policies have been designed to cope with particular problems – for example, the health risks associated with the use by cyclists of EPO, and the non-availability of medical advice to bodybuilders and others who use anabolic steroids – and it is not suggested that harm reduction policies of this kind, even if they were wholly successful in meeting their objectives within cycling and in relation to body builders, could provide an appropriate basis for dealing with the many, complex and varied problems involving drug use in sport. More specifically, insofar as these harm reduction policies have had any success – and certainly in cycling they seem to have been considerably more successful than conventional anti-doping policies in terms of controlling the use of drugs – that success appears to have been premised on some fundamental points.

The most basic of these is that the harm reduction policies and the health tests on which they are based – unlike, for example, conventional doping controls in cycling – have been accepted as legitimate by those at whom the tests are targeted. This legitimacy, in turn, appears to be based on two further considerations. The first of these is that the tests are seen as an appropriate response to what is recognised, not just by those responsible for organizing the testing but, more importantly, by the drug-using athletes themselves, as a serious health concern; in the case of cycling, this was the serious threat to the health of cyclists posed by their use of EPO and, in the case of bodybuilders, it was their lack of access to specialized medical advice to help them to deal with what they recognised as the undesirable side-effects of anabolic steroid use. Quite clearly, however, "health tests" would be much less likely to be seen as legitimate if they were designed to identify the use of drugs which, in the eyes of many people, do not pose serious health problems; the use of marijuana would be an obvious case in point. A precondition for gaining the cooperation of athletes in relation to health tests would thus seem to be that the tests address what the athletes themselves recognise as a serious health problem.

The second basis on which the harm reduction policies have been accorded legitimacy by those at whom they are targeted is that they have been framed very clearly within a non-punitive health framework, rather than within a punitive anti-doping framework. Any movement away from this health framework towards a more conventional punitive, anti-doping framework would be likely to result in the withdrawal of cooperation by the athletes concerned.

Other policy implications

Among other changes in policy, which might be considered, are two, which also affect the medical profession. The first of these relates to the fact that since the introduction of anti-doping policies in the 1960s, such policies have focused almost exclusively on the individual drug-using athlete and, as the Dubin Commission (1990:61) noted, "no effort was made to ascertain if others were involved. The obvious people – coaches, doctors, trainers – were simply ignored." This policy is unrealistic. There is now an abundance of evidence to indicate that, at least at the elite level, the drug-using athlete is normally part of a network of relationships with others, who may include team members, coaches, doctors, masseurs, trainers, managers or promoters, who are involved in supplying or administering doping substances, or in concealing their use. The highly individualistic perspective which continues to underpin the anti-doping policies of organizations such as the IOC is not only based on a misunderstanding of the social relations involved in the doping process, but it also – quite wrongly – focuses exclusively on the wrongdoing of one individual while ignoring the wrongdoing of others who are heavily implicated in the use of performance-enhancing drugs.

Professional regulation of sports medicine

There is one important area where there is scope for independent action by the medical profession, whether acting through voluntary associations such as (in Britain) the British Medical Association, through statutory bodies such as the General Medical Council or, on the international level, through organisations such as the Fédération Internationale de Médecine Sportive. Whatever decisions may be taken by the IOC and other sporting bodies in relation to doping regulations, there is clearly scope – in line with the *Lancet's* call in 1988 – for the medical profession itself to consider whether the activities of team/sports physicians are sufficiently clearly regulated. The involvement of doctors in doping clearly runs counter to the World Medical Association's declaration on principles of health care for sports medicine (WMA, 1999), and it is perhaps timely for the professional associations and regulatory bodies within the profession to give consideration to ways in which the activities of team doctors/sports physicians might be more effectively regulated and, in particular, to the conditions under which disciplinary procedures might be instigated against team doctors involved in breaching anti-doping regulations.

References

Australian Parliament (1989). Drugs in Sport: an interim report of the Senate Standing Committee on Environment, Recreation and the Arts. Commonwealth of Australia.

Black, T. (1996). "Does the ban on drugs in sport improve societal welfare?". Int. Rev. for Soc. of Sport, 31(4), 367-384.

British Medical Association Board of Science and Education (1996). *Sport and exercise medicine: policy and provision.* London, BMA.

British Medical Association (2002). *Drugs in Sport: the Pressure to Perform*, BMJ Books, London.

Brown, T. C. and Benner, C. (1984). "The nonmedical use of drugs" in W. N. Scott, B. Nisonson and J. A. Nicholas eds.: *Principles of Sports Medicine.* Baltimore, Md, and London, Williams and Wilkins, 32-39.

Coni, P., Kelland, G. & Davies, D. (1988). *AAA Drug abuse enquiry report.* Amateur Athletics Association.

Coomber, R. (1996). "The effect of drug use in sport on people's perception of sport: the policy consequences" in *The Journal of Performance Enhancing Drugs,* 1 (1), 16-20.

Cramer, R.B. (1985). "Olympic cheating: the inside story of illicit doping and the US cycling team" in *Rolling Stone*, 441, 25-26, 30.

Cycling Weekly, London, IPC Magazines Ltd.

Cycle Sport, London, IPC Magazines Ltd.

Dubin, The Honourable Charles L. (1990). *Commission of Inquiry into the Use of Drugs and Banned Practices Intended to Increase Athletic Performance.* Ottawa, Canadian Government Publishing Centre.

European Monitoring Centre for Drugs and Drug Addiction (2002). *Drugnet Europe*, No. 35, May-June, Lisbon, Portugal.

Goode, E. (1997). *Between Politics and Reason: the Drug Legalization Debate*, New York, St. Martin's Press.

Hoberman, J. (1992). *Mortal engines,* New York, Free Press.

Houlihan B. (1999). *Dying to Win: Doping in Sport and the Development of Anti-Doping Policy*, Strasbourg, Council of Europe.

Korkia, P. & Stimson, G.V. (1993). *Anabolic Steroid Use in Great Britain*, London, Centre for Research into Drugs and Health Behaviour.

"Sports medicine – is there lack of control?" in *Lancet* 1988, 2, 612.

Lenehan, P., Bellis, M. & McVeigh, J. (1996). 'A study of anabolic steroid use in the North West of England' in *The Journal of Performance Enhancing Drugs*, 1 (2), 57-70.

Millar, A.P. (1996). "Drugs in sport" in *The Journal of Performance Enhancing Drugs*, 1, (3), 106-112.

Sports Council (1996). *Doping control in the UK: a survey of the experiences and views of elite competitors, 1995*, London, Sports Council.

Todd, J. and Todd, T. (2000). "Significant events in the history of drug testing and the Olympic Movement: 1960-1999", in W. Wilson and E. Derse eds.: Doping in Elite Sport: the Politics of Drugs in the Olympic Movement, Champaign, IL, Human Kinetics, 65-128.

Voy, R. (1991). *Drugs, Sport and Politics*, Champaign, IL, Leisure Press.

Walker, C (1994) Conference Proceedings: *The 4ᵗʰ Permanent World Conference on Anti-Doping in Sport*, 5-8 September 1993, The Sports Council, London, 1994.

Waddington, I (2000). *Sport, health and drugs.* London and New York, E & F N Spon.

World Medical Association (1999). *Principles of Health Care for Sports Medicine.* 51ˢᵗ WMA General Assembly, Tel Aviv, Israel.

CHAPTER 3

THE SILENT DRAMA OF THE DIFFUSION OF DOPING AMONG AMATEURS AND PROFESSIONALS

Alessandro Donati

The history of modern sport can be traced back to the latter part of the 19th century. The history of doping covers the same period of time but has been documented in a much more fragmentary fashion. The countless people who have followed the great sporting events of the past century have generally been unaware of doping. Indeed, the alarming increase in doping that has occurred in recent decades is routinely ignored despite the doping scandals that erupt at regular intervals and threaten to destroy the very essence of sport.

In my three decades of experience in world-class sport, respectively as coach of our national teams, as the author of textbooks on the methodology of coaching, and as a sports manager, I used to believe that sporting institutions were sincere in their proclaimed desire to combat doping. But I soon started to have doubts, and eventually I realized that these institutions only had two obsessive interests: winning and exploiting sporting triumphs economically and to promote their own prestige.

For twenty years I have done everything I could to document the doping practices of which I had direct knowledge. At the same time, I must acknowledge that I was only focusing on elite sport at the top level. It only gradually occurred to me that the doping practices of elite athletes could also be affecting male and female athletes who were not yet champions but hoped to become champions some day. I eventually realized that the concept of sporting "success" was not limited to pride in victory but was far wider and more complex in scope. It could also affect the amateur athlete who aspired to outcompete his or her companions on the training field or to be admired for a more "athletic" and muscular physique.

Part one:
A long struggle against doping among high level athletes

1985: Blood transfusions are outlawed

In 1981, just a few days after I became national coach for the Italian 800m and 1500m male runners, Prof., Dr. Francesco Conconi told me that the Italian Athletics Federation had asked him to advise me about a new project. Improving upon a system used in Finland, he had developed a new system for the transfusion of selected red blood cells, in which these cells were stored at -90°, enriched with particular substances and then transfused into the athlete two or three days before an important event. "It means," he said, "an improvement of 3 to 5 seconds for 1500m races, 15 to 20 seconds for 5000m races and 30 to 40 seconds for 10,000m races."[1]. This came as a revelation to me, and I suddenly understood that doping really did exist.

I decided to tell the athletes everything. I called a meeting and described the proposal, adding that for my part, I would never accept this type of procedure, even though it had not been expressly forbidden by the IOC, because it had all the characteristics of doping. I told them they were absolutely free to choose, but that if they were to accept I would resign and go back to my desk at the Italian Olympic Committee (CONI). All seven of them said it would never occur to them to accept the use of such a technique.

Prof. Conconi waited a few weeks and then wrote to Primo Nebiolo, who was President of both the Italian Athletics Federation and the International Athletics Federation to report my lack of co-operation[2]. I was then summoned by the head coach who tried to persuade me to change my mind. I firmly refused, saying that if he wanted to perform blood transfusions on the athletes, he would first have to find another coach to replace me.

Just before the 1984 Los Angeles Olympics, Italian Athletics Federation officials became more determined; the head coach summoned my best athletes and asked them whether they wanted to improve their performances by the time of the Olympic Games by means of blood transfusions. I was present on this occasion but had been asked not to express an opinion. All seven athletes refused again. I was not even included in the Italian delegation to the Los Angeles Olympics, and immediately after the Games I was moved back to the 400m runners.

In 1985, a dear friend of mine suggested I speak to a Member of Parliament, Adriana Ceci, who was a haematologist, and she immediately took this issue to heart. Together we prepared a question in Parliament for the Minister of Health. The Minister's reply came after a few weeks: blood transfusions aimed at improving sports performances were outlawed and constituted *blood doping*[3]. The IOC promptly declared that blood transfusions were forbidden, and this method was officially designated as blood doping.

≡ Tutti devono avere il prodotti per tutto l'anno →	"Everybody should be provided with the products during the year"
— Non bisogna più utilizzare il Metiltestosterone →	"We don't have to use Metiltestosterone anymore"
— Parlarne prima del di introdurre nuovi prodotti →	"We must discuss before ingesting new products"
— Prodotti da usare: Methandrostenolone, Nerabol, OXANBP, Winstrol →	"Products to use: Methandrostenolone Nerabol Oxandrolone, Winstrol"
— I dosaggi vanno stabiliti col ett. tecnico e col prof Conconi →	"The doses must be established with the technical director"
— Strategie farmacologica in abbinamento con la strategia tecnica →	"Pharmacological strategies should be associated with technical strategies"
— seguire ogni strategia e darne copia al prof. Conconi	
— Controlli periodici ogni 20 giorni: convocazioni precise e controllo delle proteine →	"Athletes must be submitted to medical checks every twenty days"
— Cercare alternative per ridurre le dosi di anabolizzan	
⇒ Secondo prof. Conconi il 50% del risultato dipende dalla terapia III →	"Technical Director says that the 50% of the results depends on the drugs"
— Calendario dei controlli di laboratorio 12 apr.	
	6 mag
— Aumento progressivo nella stagione	22 mag → "Progressive doses increase during the season"
— Chiedere a Midule per i farmaci di sostegno	11 giu
	1 lug
	21 lug
Da 20 a 75 mg. ogni 24 giorni	10 ago
Da 80 mg a 120 mg. ogni 14 giorni	

1986: The discovery of the doping diaries

A physician and former decathlete named Daniele Faraggiana had been instructed by the Athletics Federation and by the Weightlifting Federation to "treat" the athletes of their respective national teams, mostly with anabolic steroids and with testosterone. I found Faraggiana's documents that listed everything: the names of the athletes involved, the drugs that had been administered, the respective dosages, the negative effects on their health, the performance goals that had been set, and even the "philosophy" behind the whole process[4].

It also turned out that the Anti-Doping Laboratory in Rome, duly accredited by IOC, was being used for a totally different purpose: to establish how long it would take for traces of these drugs to disappear from the athletes' urine samples. The documents also proved that Dr. Faraggiana had provided forbidden substances to Prof. Conconi, as well.

After examining these documents I thought that if I showed them to the Federation officials, saying that I would make them public if they did not dismantle the whole operation immediately, they would be easily persuaded. I soon realized just how naive I had been; they tried to prevaricate, to minimize or deny what had happened.

1987. An interview in L'Espresso

The excellent performances at the European Championships by Stephano Mei and the 400-metre runners prompted the Federation to increase the number of disciplines that were now under my supervision. I became national coach for the 100m, 200m, 400m, both relay races and the 800m.

In March, two of my sprinters, Pier Francesco Pavoni and Antonio Ullo, placed second and third in the 60m dash at the European Indoor Championships. Taking advantage of the fact that these achievements boosted my creditabillity, in August I gave an interview to *L'Espresso*, one of the major Italian magazines, in which I denounced both blood doping and the use of anabolic steroids[5]. All hell broke loose. Journalists from all over the world were already in Rome as the World Athletic Championships were about to begin. Nebiolo and his collaborators asked me to retract my comments; I replied that I would not do so.

My athletes and I were confined to a hotel in the suburbs, while the rest of the Italian team was in the town centre. No one from the Italian Athletics Federation talked to me during the Championships even though Pavoni qualified for the finals both in the 100m and in the 200m, as did the sprint relay team. The Italian Athletics Federation had already decided they were going to remove me from my position as national coach and get rid of me for good.

1989. A book titled Campioni senza Valore

I decided to record the details of this nine-year struggle in a book, *Campioni senza valore* (*Worthless Champions*), to demonstrate how the struggle had intensified and how I had encountered unimaginable levels of corruption.

The book was presented to the press in one of the major bookshops in Rome. Quite a number of journalists and other authors attended, and during the first week the sales were very good. Then, all of a sudden, the publisher stopped delivering to the bookshops and I was deluged by telephone calls and letters from all over Italy. No one could find my book. The publisher told me they were having distribution problems but that everything would be solved shortly. A few years later I learned that an international foundation had paid a large sum of money to the publisher to stop the distribution of this book.

1994. The EPO dossier

At this time I was secretary of the CONI Scientific Anti-doping Commission, so I decided to investigate the incidence of doping among professional cyclists.

I identified twelve key figures in the cycling world – athletes, physicians, officials – and assured them that the information I collected would remain strictly confidential, since my interest lay in collecting information that I would then report to the President and to the General Secretary of CONI in order to take adequate steps against doping. After four months of investigation, I arrived at some extraordinary conclusions:

1) `Anti-doping tests on cyclists seldom came out positive because they were using new substances, peptide hormones, which cannot be traced by means of urine tests.

2) In particular, the erythropoietin hormone, also known as EPO, was being used more frequently.

3) The idea of using EPO for athletes, which had evolved in endurance sports and therefore involved cyclists, had clearly come from Prof. Conconi, who had been made a member of the IOC Medical Committee some years before.

4) Prof. Conconi and his assistants had signed very important contracts with professional cycling clubs.

5) At that time the production of EPO was quite limited and was provided only to the hospitals that treated kidney disorders; this meant that the cyclists were getting it through illegal channels.

6) The cost of EPO on the black market was very high (about 150 US$ per dose); there were also other very expensive hormones, such as GH, or IGF1; in other words, the doping market was becoming as lucrative as the narcotics market.

7) Other physicians without scruples were beginning to imitate Prof. Conconi and his group, so that the use of EPO and of other peptide hormones which are undetectable via urine tests was spreading rapidly; the risk was that it would soon get completely out of hand and reach such proportions as to become attractive to the pharmaceutical companies.

I wrote a 14-page report and sent it, complete with a protocol letter, to the President and to the General Secretary of CONI. The President did not even reply. The General Secretary sent for me and said he was very concerned. I replied that CONI's behaviour was totally irresponsible and unprincipled; ever since 1980, CONI had financed Prof. Conconi's work with the athletes of various Italian national teams. Time passed but nothing more was said about my report.

1996. The EPO dossier reappears

In October 1996 one of the major Italian sports daily newspapers, *La Gazzetta dello Sport*, began a rather sterile and unenthusiastic series of articles on doping. After the sixth or seventh installment, the journalists of the *Gazzetta* met a physician in Florence, a Dr. Alessandri, who for many years had been in charge of the national women's road cycling team, and who had contributed significantly to my report.

He gave them a number of details; he also emphasized that he had already given the same details to me, nearly two and a half years before, when I was preparing a report for the President of CONI. The journalists of the *Gazzetta* came back to me asking about the report. I said: "Ask the President of CONI, I delivered it to him more than two years ago."

The President first tried to deny the existence of such a report, then admitted having received it. But he could not explain why he had kept it a secret without doing anything about it[6].

All hell broke loose again. I was in Russia for a scientific congress but my collaborators informed me of the scandal that had followed the publication of these facts, first in the *Gazzetta* and then in other newspapers. CONI was being asked to answer for:

a) having ignored the serious accusations contained in the dossier;
b) not having reported these accusations to the Court of Law;
c) not having interrupted, or even discussed, CONI's collaboration with Prof. Conconi's centres.

Many Italian and international newspapers contacted me; I was ready for the press campaign that followed, and after so many years of struggle I knew how to manage it. *L'Equipe*, the major French sports daily, dedicated front-page coverage to this issue[7].

1998. The scandal of the Rome anti-doping laboratory

In August 1998, Zdenek Zeman, coach of a first-division soccer team, *A.S. Roma*, declared in an interview that doping was widespread among soccer players. A great scandal ensued as the foreign press took up the news. Lacking any real understanding of the facts or of their significance there was a sudden and wholly superficial interest in the topic of doping, followed by an equally sudden loss of interest – boredom, perhaps – or calculated disinterest.

The Public Attorney of Turin, Raffaele Guariniello, started an investigation; he first summoned Zeman and then me on the following day. He asked me to tell him all I knew about doping among soccer players. I replied that the question should be worded differently; it should rather be: "How are anti-doping tests performed on soccer players?" During the days that followed the press reported that during my hearing I had accused the Rome Laboratory of using irregular testing procedures. The President of CONI and the president of the Sports Physicians Federation reacted violently; my declarations were false, they said, and I would lose my job at CONI unless I could prove that I was right.

And proof was found. The premises of the Rome Laboratory were searched, by order of the Public Attorney, and, as I had said, it was established that the anti-doping tests performed on soccer players did not include tests for the detection of anabolic steroids or for the other hormones[8].

The scandal became international and grew to unprecedented proportions; a number of the events that followed would prove decisive in the struggle against doping, namely:

1) The Italian government appointed a Committee of Enquiry, headed by the Vice President of the Consiglio Superiore della Magistratura, the highest judicial authority in Italy[9].

2) The Public Attorney of Turin and then the Public Attorney of Rome prosecuted the President of CONI, the President of the Sports Physicians Federation, the General Secretary of the same Federation and four technicians of the Rome Laboratory.

3) Finally, the Public Attorney of Turin forced the IOC to take notice of what was happening; the Rome Anti-doping Laboratory accredited by the IOC was closed down.

The President of CONI, Mario Pescante, who had denied the charges right to the end and accused me of lying, was found guilty by the Committee of Enquiry appointed by the Government and had to resign from office. Not long after that the General Secretary of the Sports Physicians Federation was dismissed by CONI. His dismissal was immediately followed by the President's resignation. The Laboratory technicians were found guilty by the Committee of Enquiry and dismissed.

The investigation of Prof. Conconi's twenty-year relationship with CONI suddenly moved forward as the records of his computers at the University of Ferrara were seized.

The criminal investigations of Prof. Conconi

1. The enquiry into the activities of Prof. Conconi and his colleagues began in January 1997, only a few weeks after my EPO dossier re-emerged from the archives of Mr. Pescante, the President of CONI.

2. A year and a half later, in October 1998, the Italian Carabinieri (police) searched Professor Conconi's laboratory and confiscated the files containing the results of numerous blood tests carried out on athletes active in various sports, as well as the lengthy correspondence between the Professor and the directors of the IOC, CONI and some major international sports' federations.

3. On October 26, 2000, the Public Prosecutor, Pier Guido Soprani, who had conducted a detailed investigation, asked the Judge for Preliminary Hearings for an adjournment of the trial of Prof. Conconi and certain of his colleagues[10]. At that time, he also uncovered serious implications regarding three former CONI presidents[11].

4. A few weeks later Pier Guido Soprani was transferred from the Court of Ferrara to the Court of Bologna. A new Public Prosecutor was appointed, Nicola Proto, who knew nothing of this enquiry.

5. In April 2001, before making his own decision, the Judge for Preliminary Hearings appointed a committee of experts in haematology and endocrinology to examine and draw up a report 'super partes' on the documentation confiscated from Prof. Conconi.

6. In February 2002, the committee produced a 54-page report, plus various addenda, concluding that Prof. Conconi's defence was totally groundless and could be considered as being merely an unsuccessful posterior justification[12].

7. The first of four hearings took place in March 2002; at the end of these four hearings (in May) Judge Messini decided to prosecute Prof. Conconi and his collaborators. The first hearing ended with another defeat for Conconi as the prosecution's experts easily refuted all the Professor's objections concerning their report.

8. On May 23, 2002[13], the examining judge committed Professor Conconi and two of his collaborators – Ilario Casoni and Giovanni Grazzi – to trial. The trial was held in Ferrara and began on the 29th of October 2002. Professor Conconi and his collaborators were charged with fraud in the cases of 33 athletes.
Albarello, Marco (Nordic Skiing, Olympic Champion)
Berzin, Evgeni (Cycling, winner Giro d'Italia)
Bobrik, Vladislav (Cycling)
Bontempi, Guido (Cycling)
Bugno, Gianni (Cycling, World Champion, winner Giro d'Italia)
Cecchin, Stefano (Cycling)
Cenghialta, Bruno (Cycling)
Chiappucci, Claudio (Cycling)
Chiesa, Mario (Cycling)
Damilano, Maurizio (Athletics, Olympic Champion)
Della, Bianca (Cycling)
De Zolt, Maurilio (Nordic Skiing, Olympic Champion)
Di Centa, Manuela (Nordic Skiing Olympic Champion)
Fauner, Silvio (Nordic Skiing, Olympic Champion)
Fondriest, Maurizio (Cycling, World Champion)
Frattini, Francesco (Cycling)
Furlan, Giorgio (Cycling)
Ghirotto, Massimo (Cycling)
Gotti, Ivan (Cycling, winner Giro d'Italia)
Minali, Nicola (Cycling)
Pantani, Marco (Cycling, winner Tour de France and Giro d'Italia)
Pulnikov, Wladimir (Cycling)
Polvara, G. Franco (Nordic Skiing)
Roche, Stephen (Cycling, winner Tour de France and Giro d'Italia)

Roscioli, Fabio (Cycling)
Santoromita, Antonio (Cycling)
Scaunich, Emma (Athletics)
Siboni, Marcello (Cycling)
Sørensen, Rolf (Cycling)
Ugrumov, Piotr (Cycling)
Vanzetta, Giorgio (Nordic Skiing, Olympic Champion)
Volpi, Alberto (Cycling)
Zaina, Enrico (Cycling)

Professor Conconi's collaborator, Dr. Giovanni Grazzi, former physician of the professional cycling team Carrera (which later became Mercatone Uno) was also charged with having administered doping substances. The charges were based on the "erp" files that contain a list of the dates on which EPO was administered (dosages being expressed in international units) to a number of professional cyclists.

It should be emphasized that the list above is consistent with the content of the "EPO" files. These indicate whether or not, on the date of a given blood sample, the athlete in question was being treated with erythropoietin.

It should also be emphasized that the charges against Dr. Giovanni Grazzi show that Professor Conconi was aware that one of his closest assistants was administering doping substances and was therefore helping to influence the results of major international competitions.

If the trial had indeed taken place (as we shall see, the judges accept the Defense's request to hold the trial with abbreviated procedure which is held "in camera" and is not public) it would have involved the Italian sports authorities and international sports governing bodies, in particular the IOC and UCI, since Prof. Conconi sat on the Medical Committees of both of these organizations. And if Prof. Conconi had been found guilty of administering doping substances to a large number of Italian and foreign athletes, it would have been quite an embarrassment for the IOC and the UCI to explain how it was that Prof. Conconi was asked to help them in their campaign against doping.

It is also clear that if the committee of haematology and endocrinology experts, instead of examining only the 'erp' and 'dblab' files, had also carried out a closer study of the 'EPO' files confiscated by the police and of the scientific papers presented in 1993 by Professor Conconi and his collaborators, it would clearly have been possible to establish Conconi's direct responsibility for the administration of doping substances (or) it could possibly have been possible to establish.

Indeed, both in the article published by the *International Journal of Sports Medicine* and in the paper presented by Professor Conconi at Lillehammer in August 1993, it is clearly indicated that "EPO was provided by Boheringer Biockemia, following authorization by the Medical Commission of the IOC. The hormone was administered subcutaneously in doses of 30 U/Kg of body weight, every other day for a period that ranged from 30 to 45 days."

Figure 1: 23 Athletes, but only one athlete of amatorial level (Conconi) and 22 winners of Olympic, World and European medals.

II Int. Symposium on Drugs in Sports Lillehammer, August 29-31, 1993		FERRARA UNIVERSITY July-August 1993
Conconi's lecture		**Sequestrated Conconi's files**
Detection of erythropoietin administration in sports		"EPO" File
ERYTHROPOIETIN	**Drug administered**	**ERYTHROPOIETIN**
Transferrin Receptor	**Variable considered**	**Transferrin Receptor**
23	**Subjects number (EPO treatment)**	23
148	**Samples number**	148
3.35 µg/ml	**Transferrin Receptor Average**	3.35 µg/ml
± 1.13 µg/ml	**Standard Deviation**	± 1.13 µg/ml
110	**Subjects number (for control)**	110
254	**Samples number**	254
1.91 µg/ml	**Transferrin Receptor Average**	1.91 µg/ml
± 0.45 µg/ml	**Standard Deviation**	± 0.45 µg/ml
23 ATHLETES OF AMATORIAL LEVEL		**22 ELITE ATHLETES + 1 AMATORIAL ATHLETE (Conconi)**

9. The trial began on December 5th 2002 and the judge, Valentina Tecilla, disallowed all the requests advanced by Prof. Conconi's Defense (except one as we shall see in the following ...): a) she therefore confirmed the determination of the offence of doping; b) confirmed that Prof. Conconi and his collaborators are punishable for having "favoured doping"; c) specified that, in the case of doping, the offence is punishable even when the exact date is unknown since the offence may be committed at any time before the competition; d) disallowed the request of acquittal advanced by Dr. Grazzi's Defense on the basis of the Statute of Limitations. However, the judge did allow the request advanced by Prof. Conconi's Defense to suspend proceedings because the Examining Judge had committed a formal error by slightly altering one of the charges formulated by the Public Prosecutor, Nicola Proto.

10. The judge Valentina Tecilla therefore returned all the Acts to the Examining Judge who had committed the error (an unprecedented occurrence....). In the meantime a new Examining Judge had been appointed who held on to the Acts for quite some

ALESSANDRO DONATI

time before returning them to the Public Prosecutor, Nicola Proto, who simply rewrote the charges he had already advanced two years before.

11. At long last, a new date is set for the trial: October 26th 2003. I was summoned as a witness together with other 24 persons. Just a few days before the trial, however, the summons were cancelled. The reason was that the Defense of Prof. Conconi and of his assistants advanced the request for an abbreviated procedure, involving a trial to be held "in camera" taking into account only written evidence. This request was allowed and the judge acquitted the accused because the offences were barred by the Statute of Limitations. In other words, the offences were confirmed but since the written evidence covered events only up to August 1995, they were committed outside the period of limitation. Only evidence provided by the witnesses could have shown that the offences had been committed also after said date.

12. Although seven years of investigation and prosecution had, therefore, confirmed the responsibilities of both CONI executives and of Prof. Conconi and his assistants, they all managed to avoid being convicted thanks to the Statute of Limitations.

Having started this investigation, I appear as the only loser at the end of this long battle. But in fact, the activity carried out by CONI, IOC and several International Federations in association with Prof. Conconi was definitely blocked once the judges very severely condemned their behaviour on the basis of indisputable evidence. However, the charges were dropped. It is true that ever since the beginning of the investigation (January 1997) I was constantly harassed and even today my situation within CONI is far from easy. But it is also true that having reported this situation I contributed to the beginning of a serious deliberation not only within the world of sports but also in the rest of society before it was too late; if I am not too optimistic perhaps it already is too late.

SECOND PART:
THE SILENT DRAMA OF THE DIFFUSION OF DOPING AMONG AMATEURS AND PROFESSIONALS

While these events were taking place, while I continued my struggle against doping among high-level athletes, I gradually became aware of a new phenomenon: the increasing diffusion of doping among intermediate-level athletes and even among amateur and junior athletes.

I soon understood that this was a serious situation both from an ethical standpoint and regarding the health-related risks involved. Elite athletes do indeed play perilous games with doping substances, but as much as possible, they are careful to keep the more danger-ous side-effects under control by means of accurate medical and laboratory tests.

If amateur athletes resort to doping, they may easily take megadoses or take these substances for too long, thereby making the health-related risks even greater.

Evaluation of the Dimensions of the Doping Phenomenon

The dimensions of the phenomenon can be assessed according to the following four factors:

1) Illegal commerce and seizure of doping substances
2) Sale of drugs having a doping potential
3) Results of surveys on awareness and possible consumption of doping substances
4) Results of anti-doping urine tests

1) Illegal Commerce and Seizure of Doping Substances

In Italy as well as abroad, a barrage of news reports about the confiscation of doping drugs, the ongoing police investigations and court cases, and the abnormal increase in the sales of drugs useful in 'doping' contexts were broadcast on a daily basis. All of this helped to show the public the extent to which even amateurs were making use of doping products to boost their athletic abilities and "improve" their physiques.

This information enables us to define a phenomenon of extremely worrying dimen-sions, a phenomenon that is growing continually and that involves all countries with a high potential for consuming these drugs. Its reverberations seem to be strongest in countries such as Italy, Sweden, Belgium and France, where the judiciary and the police have done the most to discourage such practices (unlike in other countries that have underestimated or even deliberately ignored the problem).

The Italian data on the increasing number and volume of drug confiscations carried out over the last four years have brought to light a vast phenomenon of illegal traffic on an international scale. At the same time, it turns out that in almost all of the countries where such traffic was found to be rife, no legal or judicial actions aimed at prevention or suppression were initiated.

Confiscations of potential doping drugs have been carried out on an almost daily basis by the police and confirm the results of surveys carried out in Italy by several mar-ket research institutes that have, from time to time, decided to investigate the problem, interviewing large cross-sections of the general population on both the inclination to take such drugs and on their actual consumption. These research questionnaires, even though they have not been administered systematically, have enabled us to document and catalogue the scale and type of doping practices that are currently in use.

Our portrait of the quantitative scale of this phenomenon, emerging from the legal investigations and the market surveys, is supplemented by data regarding the sales of the main pharmaceutical drugs that can be used for doping purposes[14]. From these data, an alarming but illuminating picture emerged concerning the huge volume of sales of certain pharmaceutical products of a hormonal nature, both in Italy and around the world, that can be used for doping, including erythropoietic and growth hormones. These sales, as we will see in the following paragraphs, greatly exceed the actual need for such drugs given the numbers of legitimate patients for whom they are supposedly manufactured.

Produced by the big multinational manufacturers, the drugs that can be used for doping pass in various ways into the hands of traffickers and then end up being distributed at the retail level (in many cases by drug dealers who mix them together with other kinds of drugs), thus reaching the consumer. Recently, however, this system has been complicated due to the gradual entry into the international market of a large number of small and medium-sized pharmaceutical companies located in several former Soviet republics, Asia, South America and even Africa[15].

As has already been noted, the confiscation of doping drugs represents an important index of the spread of this phenomenon. An index that is even more significant if we consider that the police and magistrates have, up until recently, been operating without any specific legal framework, motivated instead by personal initiative originating in their awareness of the problem, but thus operating with limited resources in turn limiting their investigations.

It should be added that investigators often come across cases of doping drugs quite by accident, during enquiries into the trafficking of traditional drugs. Among the drugs confiscated from traffickers they may also find anabolic steroids or growth hormones, erythropoietin, testosterone, IGF1, blood derivatives or other doping drugs.

The following analysis has been limited to major drug confiscations in Italy over the five and a half year from June 1997 to December 2002. The specific seizures included in the analysis have been chosen due to their significant quantity and commercial value or due to the paticular kind of drug trafficking that brought them to light. For an extensive overview, please see Appendix A.

Table 1: Illegal commerce and seiszure of doping substances in Italy.

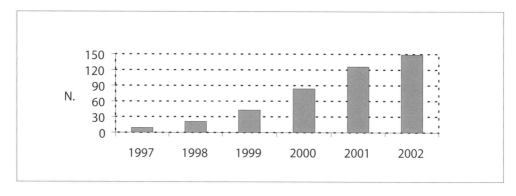

The enormous increase in this phenomenon can be observed in the diagram above which shows the confiscation of drugs reported by various information media[16]. However, it must be remembered that we often do not hear about the discovery or confiscation of small or medium quantities of drugs. Either because these operations form part of much larger and more complex operations and only represent one particular stage in a police enquiry, or simply because the police do not always choose to release the information to the press for reasons having to do with their methods of investigation. Above all, it must be noted that the drugs sold illegally for doping purposes and those that the police do manage to confiscate represent only a tiny percentage (not more than 2%) of all the illegal drugs actually on the market.

Given this enormous increase in doping practices among the various categories of amateur athletes, we must ask ourselves about the reasons for such behaviour. Once we understand that the world of sports, particularly in individual disciplines, is driven by a continual striving to achieve ever higher performances, to the point where any ethical consideration has to take second place, it becomes easier to understand how the increase in doping practices has evolved. When core members of a particular sport (and by that I mean the people – athletes, coaches and managers – who occupy the principal roles in top-class sport) have decided that their one and only goal is to improve performance at any cost, a chain reaction starts which consequently affects the whole environment of that particular sport and dictates how the performances can be achieved. The whole system now moves towards a doping crisis. At this point the tendency toward unbridled competition inexorably spreads down to the base of the pyramid and eventually becomes the rule rather than the exception.

Doping has thus spread in stages from world-class to amateur sporting circles and then down to local gymnasiums until, as we have seen, it results in a great deal of illegal trafficking that supplements the existing traffic in narcotics. Through international police cooperation, we now confront the necessity of building up a centralized data bank that can identify the actors and provide a better understanding of the criminal organizations involved in Italy and around the world.

ALESSANDRO DONATI

2) Sale of Drugs with a Doping Potential

Covering sales that had taken place in 1997. The first official data representing sales of drugs in Italy that can also be used for doping purposes were published in August 1998 by Italy's leading financial daily newspaper *Il Sole 24 Ore*. The article listed the different kinds of drugs involved, including the erythropoietic hormone (or EPO), the somatotropic hormone (or GH), anabolic steroids, stimulants, beta-blockers and other kinds of drugs. The market value based on official sales of such drugs was in excess of 250 million euros, but certain distinctions need to be made[17].

a) A considerable proportion of the total, over 100 million euros, covered sales of somatotropic and erythropoietic hormones; however, a distinction must be made between their use by athletes for doping purposes and their therapeutic use in the treatment of certain important pathological conditions. However the medical uses of anabolic steroids are very limited, leading to the assumption that almost all sales of these drugs can be ascribed to doping.

b) It can therefore be calculated that, in Italy, official sales in 1997 of drugs used for doping purposes reached around 150 million euros. Moreover, this estimate is confirmed by the magistrates' enquiries that took place mostly in Piedmont, Lazio and Sicily, which brought to light the following facts: a) many false doctors' prescriptions (in Piedmont alone it was found that out of a total of 112,000 prescriptions examined around 60,000 were not genuine) were enabling athletes to obtain drugs for doping, even at the expense of the Italian national health system; and b) systematic thefts of doping drugs were found to have been made from pharmaceutical stores.

c) From 1998 to the present day, official sales of drugs with doping potential have increased disproportionately year by year; for example, sales of erythropoietin have been increasing by 30% per year, rising from 60 million euros in 1997 to around 78 million euros in 1998 and 100 million euros in 1999; sales of growth hormone have increased on average by 25% per year, going from 55 million euros in 1997 to 67 million in 1998 and 83 million in 1999[18].

d) At the end of 2000, official statistics on sales in Italy of important drugs with doping potential were finally published, thanks to work conducted by the Ministry of Health's national observatory on medicines. Research was based on the examination of 181 million prescriptions collected from around 16,000 pharmacies belonging to the Federfarma association. The data collected in the first half of the year 2000, revealed that erythropoietin and growth hormone headed the list of the drugs that had sold the most in Italy; it is disconcerting to note that their sales volumes increased further to reach 79 million euros for erythropoietine and 54 million euros for growth hormone, representing a final estimate for the year 2000 of 158 million euros spent on erythropoietin and 108 million euros on growth hormone[19].

Table 2: Official sale of EPO and GH in Italy.

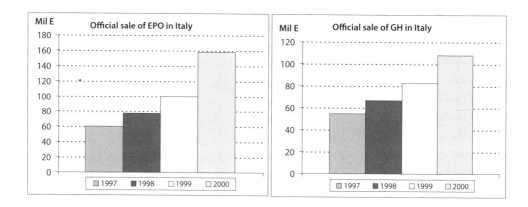

e) We must also add to this total the enormous quantity of doping drugs bought by Italian athletes in the pharmacies of neighbouring countries, particularly Switzerland. It is almost impossible to calculate the amount of drugs bought abroad by Italian customers, but the magistrates' investigations mentioned above would seem to indicate that the figures are extremely high; for example, in a single enquiry carried out by the well-known Swiss magistrate Carla Del Ponte, a former close associate of Giovanni Falcone in his investigations into the Mafia's role in drug trafficking, the evidence showed that over a million doses of stimulants, amounting to several million euros, were sold illegally to two Italians involved in the world of amateur cycling[20].

f) We must also take into account the enormous volume of sales realized through 1) the so-called thefts carried out in pharmaceutical warehouses as mentioned above; 2) illegal imports by criminal groups; 3) illegal purchases made through the Internet; and 4) the illegal production by clandestine laboratories in Italy. On the basis of the large, but nevertheless random and fragmentary, number of confiscations carried out in Italy, the volume of illegal sales can be estimated to at least 330 million euros.

g) Therefore, if we add illegal sales of drugs with doping potential to "official" sales, and if we estimate that this latter category increases by 30% a year, then the estimated 150 million euros in 1997 must have increased to at least 335 million euros in 2002, bringing total sales of doping drugs to Italian customers to an estimated total of around 665 million euros.

h) This figure does not, however, include the large annual volume of "supplement" sales, in particular the branched-chain amino acids and creatine that, based on a series of data, can be valued at 1,600 million euros minimum. This estimate also includes the growing spread of such supplements among preadolescents and young teenagers, as shown in a recent investigation carried out by the Rome municipality among about 12,000 middle school pupils (11-13 years old) in the capital. This sample group was well-balanced, representing a total of around 95,000 pupils, and the results showed that about 10% of the pupils took protein supplements[21]. A previous study carried out in Milan yielded similar results[22].

Therefore, all Italian athletes, subdivided into medium-level or top-level, young practitioners and amateurs, spend around 2,500 million euros per year on drugs and substances purporting to increase their sporting capacities or, for some, to improve their physiques. Other products widely consumed by athletes, such as homeopathic or herbal products, multi-vitamins, mineral or iron supplements, or even vegetable-based hormones and other special "supplements" whose properties are often carelessly advertised as being beneficial, even for neuro-muscular co-ordination, have not been included in this calculation.

Consider, for example, that Federsalus, an association of a few companies marketing "energy" products and tonics, had already announced in 1998 that sales in Italy had reached 78 million packages with a monetary value of over 550 million euros[23]. As the growth rate in sales is around 15 million per annum, the volume of sales in this category of supplements could easily have reached the one billion euro mark by 2002.

Many of these products, as we have seen from the many confiscations carried out in Italy, are not even registered with the Ministry of Health and are, therefore, sold under totally illegal conditions. As already mentioned, in many cases it has even been found that these products also contained doping substances. It goes without saying that a volume of business on this scale can exert a considerable influence in promoting the different kinds of supplements available on the market well beyond their actual therapeutic or dietary advantages – assuming there are any – even to the point of intimidating those who oppose their use.

In 1998, the Finnish university in Jyväskylä estimated the volume of sales of drugs with doping potential worldwide at around 18 billion euros; in 2002 this figure could have reached at least 30 billion euros. For example, according to a study published in the French newspaper "Le Monde," worldwide sales of erythropoietin alone reached around 4 billion euros in 2000, bringing sales of this hormone to second place in global drug sales. Also according to "Le Monde", only about a sixth of EPO sales was destined for patients with pathological conditions that require their use, while the remaining five- sixths were bought by athletes[24]. However, there are good reasons to believe that the estimated volume of sales of EPO cited by this French newspaper is on the low side. In fact, the American multinational Amgen declared that, for 2003, sales of erythropoietin (marketed under the brand name of Epogen) and darbepoetin (marketed under the brand name of Aranesp) reached an annual estimate of around 5 billion euros[25]. In conclusion, the realities of the estimate of 30 billion euros of sales worldwide in doping drugs, both legal and illegal, stems from the single case of illegal traffic between England and Belgium[26], only a fraction of which is intercepted by the police. A fraction, however, amounting to around 1.2 billion euros. If we add to this another case of illegal trafficking intercepted in January 2002 in Austria[27], we can already see that there is no link between the two cases, as there is no evidence of any link between either of these cases and the big investigation carried out subsequently in Bologna. This diversification in the sources of the trafficking shows that, unfortunately, the estimate of 30 billion euros is more than likely to be accurate.

Moreover, if we add worldwide sales of drugs with doping potential to sales of so-called supplements, we end up with astronomical figures, approaching 100 billion euros. Just consider, as an example, that in June 2000 the European Commission had imposed fines totalling 115 million euros on five companies charged with having created a worldwide cartel to control prices of a single amino acid, Lysine[28]. Yet another example can be found in United States sales of a so-called supplement called DHEA (a hormone which is regarded as a precursor of testosterone) that in 2002 reached a level of 8 billion euros in sales. It is also significant that sales of androstenedione, another purported testosterone precursor, increased dramatically in the United States after a famous baseball player (Mark McGwire) admitted that he had taken the substance to boost his energy level.

3) Results of Surveys on Awareness and possible Consumption of Doping Substances

Only recently has the social significance of the doping phenomenon been recognized, first in the United States and then also in Europe. While there have been some surveys that track the consumption of doping drugs, we still do not have a clear picture of the actual dimensions of this enormous submerged consumer market.

The only official national investigation that has taken place in Italy on doping practices was a survey carried out in 1989 by the Doxa Institute at the request of CONI in the wake of a scandal that involved several sports. This survey covered 1,015 athletes from 16 different sporting disciplines, and it was found that around 10% of top-level Italian athletes used some kind of doping drug. The results also showed that 7% of them said they took doping drugs through blood transfusions[29].

The Italian Ministry of Defence carried out a study in 1994 on no fewer than 35,000 eighteen-year-olds who were examined at the time of their induction into military service. This survey showed that 2% (or about 700 young men) used anabolic steroids[30]. If we consider that not even half of the boys examined were engaged in any sport at all, we can deduce that at least 4% of those practicing a sport used anabolic steroids. These data are particularly alarming if we consider that they date back nine years and if we take into account the fact that anabolic steroids are only one possible form of doping.

A study carried out in 1999 at the University of Padua on a sample of 3,768 young people between ten and twenty-three years old showed that, out of the 2,562 people who practiced some sport, around 5% used doping drugs[31]; in order of popularity these were amphetamines, anabolic steroids, erythropoietin and growth hormone. Considering the wide age range of this group and the very low risk of doping in the lower age group, we have to conclude that the percentage of older subjects (those from 18 to 23

Table 3: Percentage of young people (under 23) using doping drugs.

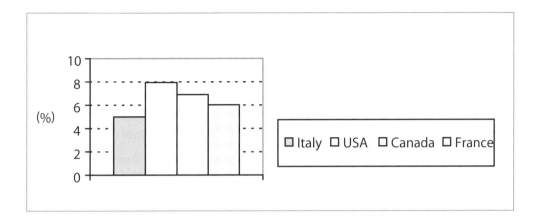

years old) using doping drugs is considerably higher and therefore comparable to data from other industrialized countries.

In the United States a research study was carried out by means of a questionnaire administered to adolescent students regarding their use of growth hormone. The result was that 2.86% of the students answered in the affirmative. The same study revealed that 65% of the students who used growth hormones had also used anabolic steroids[32]. A number of studies carried out in several different countries indicate that these drugs are in widespread use among teenagers; in the United States, around 3% of 14-16 year-olds are users[33] and percentages of between 1 and 3 have also been found to be users in three Canadian studies[34], two Swedish studies[35], two South African studies[36], one British study[37] and one Australian study[38].

On the basis of the estimated volumes being bought and sold illegally, and as confirmed by survey results, we can hypothesize that Italians who use doping drugs, whether they are athletes who belong to the sports federations, amateur athletes or ordinary citizens frequenting body-building gyms, total altogether around 400,000 people. This calculation is derived from the assumed national expenditures in this area, estimated to be around 580 million euros (based on official sales and estimated illegal sales of drugs with doping potential) and an average per capita per annum expenditure of about 1,600 euros on the purchase of doping drugs[39].

A wide-ranging research study carried out by the Rome municipality among teenage pupils between 14 and 19 years of age demonstrated the existence of a particularly close relationship between consumption of doping drugs and consumption of protein supplements such as creatine and amino acids[40].

In fact, the proportion of doping-substance users among consumers of protein supplements is a good 10 times higher than among non-consumers.

Table 4: Declared creatine/aminoacids and doping substances consumption.

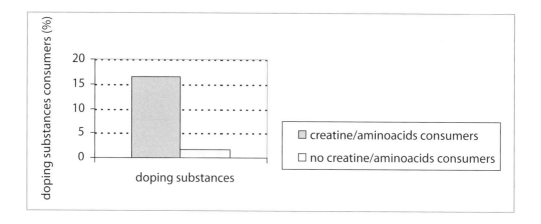

Another research study carried out in the Rome area among 11 to 13 year old pupils demonstrated that there is a strong correlation between consumers of protein supplements and consumers of pharmaceutical products based on vitamins and minerals[41].

Here, too, the proportion of amino acid users among those who consume vitamin- and mineral-based pharmaceutical products is ten times greater than among non-consumers. The same result was obtained for creatine users; there are eight times as many creatine users among consumers of vitamin- and mineral- based products than among non-consumers.

These data also highlight the importance of correct dietary education and information in preventing doping. All of this shows that the unjustified use of protein sup-

Table 5: Declared creatine/aminoacids and vitamins/minerals consumption.

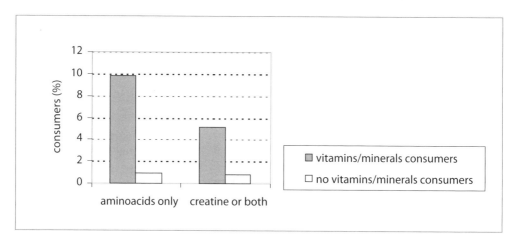

ALESSANDRO DONATI

plements can, in fact, serve as a factor that predisposes subjects to the use of doping substances.

4) Results of Anti-Doping Urine Tests

Among the 400,000 Italians who probably use doping substances, official anti-doping tests result in only 150 positive cases per year. This limited number of cases depends, mainly, on the extremely limited number of athletes targeted by the anti-doping tests which are aimed at a particularly narrow sample of federation-affiliated athletes (estimated at around 0.1 – 0.2%). However, this is also related to the limitations of the testing methods.

In fact, even extrapolating the current testing system to all athletes at all levels, we would still run the risk of testing only 12,000 of the estimated 400,000 users of doping substances.

This observation highlights the inadequacy of the anti-doping tests as a solution to the problem, particularly with reference to the vast world of amateur and youth sports. Allthough it is extremely expensive and difficult to put into operation, ideally, it should be up to the sports institutions and centres to develop an anti-doping system as these are at least nominally interested in preventing and eliminating doping among high-level athletes. But it should also be clear that the anti-doping tests, because they are intrusive and because of their high cost, cannot possibly represent a practical solution for the prevention of doping in the practice of amateur and youth sporting activities. Moreover, truly effective testing would require a complex organizational network which cannot be set up for basic sports activities.

THIRD PART:
CRIMINAL INVESTIGATIONS IN THE GYMNASIUMS

After I testified in January 1997 (my hearing lasted from 10:00 am to 2:00 on the following day), the Public Prosecutor of Arezzo, Giovanni Scolastico, began a long investigation which lead to two separate investigations which were later developed by other prosecutors: one in Ferrara concerning Prof. Conconi that was carried out by Pier Guido Soprani; and the other in Bologna, carried out by Giovanni Spinosa, regarding doping among cyclists and the activities of an important pharmacy.

The Bologna investigation, carried out by Giovanni Spinosa, lead to the wire-tapping of wholesale dealers of doping substances, which in turn lead to the discovery of a network of dealers who sold these substances to gymnasiums. The result of 18 months of investigation was impressive; it traced an illegal trade in doping substances worth over 20 million euro. The magistrate ordered the arrest of 41 persons and confirmed the involvement of criminal organizations, in particular the Neapolitan camorra[42]. The investigation revealed that many gymnasiums are directly involved in the use of doping substances and in the distribution of these to other sports; the weekly amount (for each gymnasium) was estimated to be about 1000-2000 doses a week (including anabolic steroids, testosterone, growth hormone erythropoietin, various types of stimulants, etc.). Similar investigations, although not quite as extensive, were carried out by prosecutors in other Italian cities: the major ones were carried out in Rome, Naples, Palermo, Cagliari, Turin: Padova, Trani, Viterbo, Genoa, Latina, Aosta, Milan, Brescia, Como, Venice, Florence, Pistoia, Udine, Trento, Pesaro, Salerno, Reggio Emilia, Catania, Savona, Lecco, Imperia, Bolzano, Rovereto, Varese, Piacenza, Ancona and Modena.

Each one of these investigations showed that behind the doping among elite athletes innumerable daily tragedies, involving hundreds of thousands of amateur athletes and body builders, occur out of sight and are ignored by everyone.

I doubt that this happens only in Italy. My country is hardly transparent in this regard, but at least over the past few years public prosecutors and the police have become aware of the issue. It is true that each prosecutor works on his own and does not inform his colleagues who are investigating similar situations, which means that the results of the investigations are never complete. Yet it must be said that in Italy the criminal courts and the police are directly involved in the struggle against doping.

I seldom hear of similar investigations in other European countries. Most of the foreign journalists I know tell me they have not heard about police investigations into the illegal commerce of doping substances in their countries.

The Italian investigations show that, in addition to the multinational pharmaceutical manufacturers, there are now a number of small and medium-sized companies in Eastern Europe, Asia and South America involved in the production and illegal sale of enormous quantities of drugs that will be used for doping and in stock farming. All these substances are sent wherever there is enough money to pay for them.[43] How can we believe that large amounts do not end up in gymnasiums all over Europe?

The basic information deriving from the Bologna investigation has made possible an understanding of the actual scope of the doping practices that have spread among amateur athletes. We now know something about the characteristics of the people who make up this world, the volume of business generated, the international spread of trafficking, and the partial compromising of major public institutions. It is a social problem of considerable dimensions, and what is more, a problem that is destined to grow, at least over the next several years.

People involved in the Bologna Investigation

Our understanding of the mechanisms underlying the spread of doping among the clients of gymnasiums and amateur sports enthusiasts; the cultural and psychological characteristics of the people involved; the conversational style and type of language used among traffickers and suppliers of doping drugs – all of this is illuminated by the transcripts of conversations intercepted by the Carabinieri narcotics squad during an operation carried out at the request of the Bologna Public Prosecutor's office. Please see Appendix B for the extensive details.[44]

101 different pharmaceutical products were confiscated during the investigation:
43 drugs based on anabolic steroids; 27 drugs containing peptide hormones (growth hormone, gonadotropin, erythropoietin, gonadorelin); 19 drugs containing stimulants (caffeine, ephedrine, amphetamine); 12 miscellaneous drugs (antiestrogen, hepato protective, etc).

The illegal traffic in the above-mentioned products involved the following 15 countries: Argentina, Australia, Egypt, France, Holland, Germany, Greece, Italy, Portugal, Czech Republic, Rumania, Russia, Spain, Turkey, USA.

119 gymnasiums were involved in the investigations. The commercial value amounts to 19 million euro.

In order to gain a better understanding of the complex organization of the illegal doping drug trade we can use as an illustration the sales and purchases made during a given week by one of the wholesalers involved in the investigation.

Figure 3: Statistics regarding the investigation.

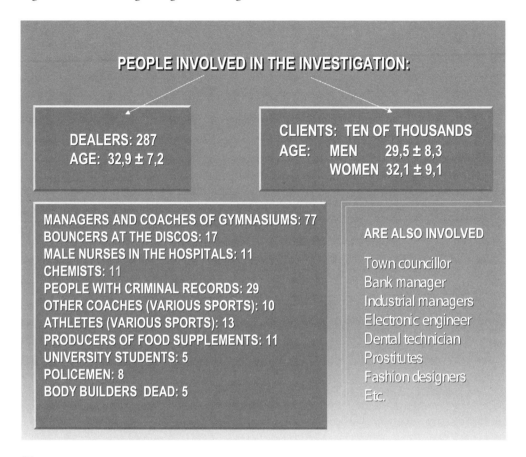

FOURTH PART:
CAUSES OF THE DIFFUSION OF DOPING

Whereas a series of factors occurring within the world of sport constitute the origin of the doping problem, some outside factors have also contributed to the complexity and scope of this problem.

Causes within the World of Sports

The first and most important cause is the uninhibited ambition to exceed individual and absolute limits. This is the concept promoted by the sports system as its dominant frame of reference. The sports system thus ignores the risks involved in focusing exclusively on quantitative limits as opposed to qualitative aspects of the sports experience.

ALESSANDRO DONATI

Figure 4: Sales and purchaces.

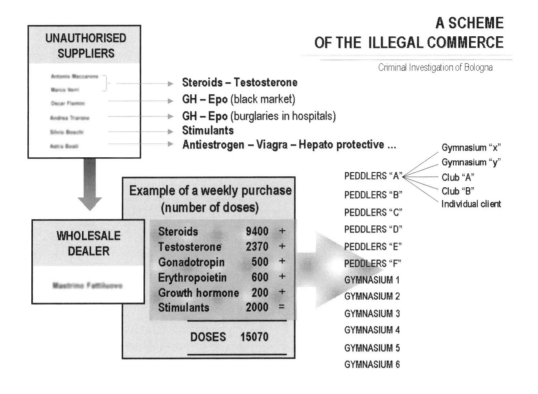

As a result, sport has become an excessive striving towards quantitative and therefore alienating limits.

Unregulated professionalization of roles. This phenomenon has affected a number of sports and has involved not only the athletes but above all managers, coaches and doctors. From the 1970s onwards, this trend has developed throughout western Europe and has been encouraged by the replacement of volunteer sports officials with professionals.

This situation developed due to the increasing commercial value of sporting activities and out of the desire to do something about the predominance that the eastern European countries had enjoyed for many years. These countries had invested heavily in the world of sports, both financially and by creating a professional organization that was capable of maximizing the motivation and talent of young athletes and, in particular, of promoting the development of world-class athletes.

The changes the western European countries underwent were, however, dissimilar[45]. They also changed the value system by emphasizing a frenetic drive towards success. This led the managers within the central organization of sporting federations to increasingly rely on a narrow group of professional collaborators, skilled experts and medical specialists who were motivated to obtain the best performances possible from the athletes under their management in order to justify their own positions and privileges. The rest of the sporting world – the volunteers – have gradually fallen into line with these political and organizational tendencies that: a) have transformed the organization of sport for young people into straightforward talent recruitment; b) have taken control of world-class athletes, wooing them away from the clubs in which they were first developed; and c) have subverted respect for fundamental ethical and educational principles, subordinating them to the pursuit of success.

Amateurs tend to emulate elite athletes. How prominent athletes behave and reach stardom becomes, in both positive and negative aspects (including the practice of doping), the point of reference for young aspiring athletes who are eager to emulate their sporting heroes. This means that the practice of doping has gradually become embedded at all levels, starting with the highest and percolating right down to the ranks of the most casual amateurs.

The crisis of sports ethics. This crisis has developed out of the behaviours that have already been described and whose gradual spread has brought about a systematic flouting of the basic rules of sports ethics. Because appropriate sanctions are not always imposed on the guilty parties, there is a widespread sense of mistrust demoralizing managers and coaches in some sports to the point where they simply abandon the world of sport altogether.

At this point the sports system does not seem to fully understand the extent to which it has distanced itself from its own ethical principles to the point where, in the eyes of some outside observers, it has lost much of its legitimacy as means of educating young people. This confusion in the sports system has been symbolized by its passive acceptance of the doping phenomenon. It is significant that it was institutions outside the world of sports that first brought this problem to light and tried to limit its spread. At the same time, the sports institutions have denied or minimized the phenomenon, or condemned it in a general way, being primarily concerned about deflecting suspicion and accusations onto other parties, while opposing and isolating anyone who criticizes their behaviour.

Distortion of youth sports. This is the logical consequence of what we have seen above. It began with the national sporting federations insisting on children becoming members of federations at ever younger ages. Then it was aggravated by operational programmes that were oriented towards the selection of children who were thought to have talent, with the result that children who were not considered sufficiently talented were relegated to the sidelines. This distortion reached its apex as a system of precocious specialization was instituted for the youngest children wanting to practice a particular sport. And, as this system in turn lead to an excessive increase in the frequency and level of training, coaching, practice sessions and competition, thus greatly reducing or eliminating altogether any aspect of "fun" in the practice og sports for children. This exasperation also led to a high proportion of children abandoning sports at an early age due to its monotony and ruthless selection procedures.

Causes outside the World of Sports

Among the causes for the spread of doping originating outside the world of sport we can identify the following:

National political interests. From the 1960s onward, sport was a means by which many countries, and especially those belonging to the former Soviet republics, tried, for reasons having to do with both domestic and international politics, to project a positive image and gain respect in the rest of the world through the exceptional performances of their athletes.

In these countries doping was organized at the government level; a fact documented by previously confidential documents and testimonies emerging from state archives and halls of justice.

Starting in the 1970s, some countries opposing the communist bloc were however organizing something very similar in a centralized fashion, in order to become more competitive in international sport. Two decades later it is clear that the doping of elite athletes played its own role in the Cold War (see Spitzer in this volume).

Even today it still seems that certain political leaders in eastern Europe have not changed their thinking, judging by what the current President of the Russian Republic, Vladimir Putin, recently declared: "Sporting triumphs can bring more harmony to a nation than a hundred political slogans."

Commercial interests of the pharmaceutical companies. This is an important factor we should try to understand. First of all, it should be noted how, in the eastern bloc countries, the practice of doping was limited to enhancing the performance of top-level athletes. In the absence of other motives to spread this practice to other athletes, it was indeed understood in these countries that the practice of doping was a special procedure reserved for a select few and was to be kept out of reach of ordinary citizens.

In countries lacking an industrial or commercial system of a private nature, there was no motivation to produce doping drugs for the 'ordinary' citizen. This is contrary to what has happened in the more industrialized countries, where a few small pharmaceutical manufacturers, often clandestine, began producing those drugs that are most in demand for doping purposes. Now they see the potential for a substantial market among athletes. When the major multinational pharmaceutical companies recognized the potential for commercial development, and having the ability to penetrate any market effectively, they began to take over the production and distribution of these drugs. In the next phase, which is underway, many small and medium-sized pharmaceutical companies, most of them based in some of the former Soviet republics and in Asia, have entered this market, thereby further complicating an already serious situation on an international scale.

The medicalisation of society: this is a phenomenon that is characteristic of countries that enjoy a higher standard of living and that eliminated malnutrition, hygienic problems and epidemics long ago. Now, however, they find themselves faced with the other side of the coin, the negative aspects of an enormous flood of drugs on the market deriving from the manufacturers' incessant desire to increase their turnover.

For example, a growing number of drugs have been made available to the public for the relief of physical pain or psychological discomfort, many of which can be bought without a prescription, while others often find that it is no problem at all to find a doctor willing to write a prescription for the drug in question. The increasing availability of such products has undoubtedly contributed to an improvement in many people's quality of life. However, it has also led to growing abuse in that many people take them even for minor ailments (see Waddington in this volume).

Such products are now considered to be normal, both by those who prescribe or recommend them and by those who consume them. Here is how the effects of growth hormone are described by a company based in the Bahamas, which sells the drug over the Internet:

> "It rejuvenates you, enables you to lose 14% of your body fat within six months, increases your muscle mass by 9%, improves your athletic performance, enhances sexual capacity, reduces stress levels, increases immunity to disease, decreases blood pressure and cholesterol levels, promotes new hair growth, eliminates cellulite, treats cardiac problems, eliminates osteoporosis, renews the skin, increases memory capacity and cognitive functions, improves sleep, stimulates neurons, improves eyesight, etc."

Other economic interests. These include the sponsors who draw up contracts with elite athletes, with club teams, national teams, national and international sporting federations, national and international Olympic committees and with the organizers of various sporting events. It is obvious that the sponsors invest money in sports for the purpose of gaining publicity advantages, and it is equally obvious that such advantages derive from the performances of the athletes who are sponsored. This is why the sponsors are interested in the success of the athletes and, consequently, in anything that might improve their performances. And this despite the fact that investment in publicity may be compromised by serious cases of doping that are attributed to their athletes.

We must also consider the interests of the networks that buy the television rights to the most important sporting events. (From 1997 to the present day, the total number of hours that television around the world has dedicated to sporting events has doubled.)

Needless to say, these broadcasters have the same interest as their sporting partners in obtaining the highest profit possible from these events.

Finally, there are the economic interests of the organizers of major sporting competitions: international meetings, national championships, continental championships, world championships, Olympic games, etc. For example, the IOC received 700 million dollars just for the television rights to broadcast the Sydney Games in the United States, and a further 600 million dollars for the broadcasting rights in the rest of the world. It also received 550 million dollars from global sponsors and around 600 million dollars from several other sources, for a total revenue of close to 2.5 billion dollars. The FIFA football federation and the organizers of the 2002 World Football Championship received over 800 million euros just for the television rights[46].

As already stated; by signing contracts with the athletes or the sporting organizations to which they belong, each of these economic operators, are working towards the same goal: optimum results. Now doping, too, has become one of the factors in the planning of sporting successes.

Notes

1 Donati A., Campioni senza valore, 26; Ponte alle Grazie Firenze, 1989.

2 Donati A., Campioni senza valore, 32-33, lettera del 10-06-1983; Ponte alle Grazie Firenze, 1989.

3 Italia, Ministero della Sanità. Decreto ministeriale 31-05-1985.

4 Donati A., Campioni senza valore, 74-85; Ponte alle Grazie Firenze, 1989.

5 Gallucci C., Droga per la vittoria, L'Espresso, 120-123, 30-08-1987.

6 Bondini G., Piccioni V., Un medico denuncia:dilaga il doping, La Gazzetta dello Sport, 25, 25-10-1996.
Bergonzi P., Bondini G., Piccioni V., Riaperta dal CONI l'inchiesta doping, La Gazzetta dello Sport, 25, 26-10-1996.
Bondini G., Piccioni V., Dossier-Donati: catenaccio del CONI, La Gazzetta dello Sport, 23, 29-10-1996.

7 Roger G., Le terrible dossier, L'Equipe, 1-3, 14-01-1997.

8 Attorney's Office of Torino, Minutes of the preliminary hearing of Donati A., Civolani C., 25-08-1998.

9 Report of the Commission of Inquiry, established by W.Veltroni, Minister of Sports, 10-10-1998.

10 Attorney's Office of Ferrara, Closure of the preliminary inquiry and contextual notice of action. 25-10-2000. Assistant Public Prosecutor Soprani P.G.

11 Attorney's Office of Ferrara, Request for partial dismissal. 25-10-2000. Assistant Public Prosecutor Soprani P.G.

12 Court of Ferrara Proc. 9580/99. Expert's report by Banfi G., D'Onofrio G., Judge Messini D'Agostini P., 12-02-2002.

13 Court of Ferrara, Department of the Judges for preliminary inquiries and hearings, Judgement. Judge Messini D'Agostini P, 23-05-2002.

14 Italy, Department for the supervision and evaluation of drugs.

15 Indictment for illegal trade of hormones and substances having an anabolic effect destined to doping procedures in humans. Bologna, 21-06-2000.

16 Comune di Roma, Dipartimento Cultura-Sport, Campagna di informazione e sensibilizzazione sul problema del doping, 2003.
   Italia, Ministero della Pubblica Istruzione, Prevenire il doping tra gli studenti, Manuale per gli insegnanti, 2001.
17 Grassia F., Il Sole 24 ore, 10-08-1998.
18 Grassia F., Il Sole 24 ore, 10-08-1998.
   Italy, Department for the supervision and evaluation of drugs.
19 Italy, Ministry of Health, The use of drugs in Italy, National Report I Semester 2000.
20 Chili di amfetamine per ciclisti italiani, Corriere del Ticino, 15-06-1996
21 Comune di Roma, Dipartimento Cultura-Sport, Campagna di informazione e sensibilizzazione sul problema del doping, 2003.
22 ANSA: 17-06-2000.
23 ANSA: 26-10-1999.
24 Lorelle V., La substance vedette de l'industrie biotechnologique, Le Monde, 11-05-1999.
25 Amgen INC, Report 2003, Management's discussion and analysis of financial condition and results of operations.
26 ANSA: 23-07-2002.
   Saise record de steroides anabolisants, Le Soir en ligne, 24-07-2002.
27 ANSA: 26-01-2002.
28 ANSA: 07-06-2000.
29 ANSA: 13-12-1989.
30 ANSA: 10-03-1997.
31 Stucchi E., Sondaggio tra i baby sportivi: uno su dieci ricorre al doping, Corriere della Sera, 17, 23-11-1999.
32 Rickert VI, Pawlak-Morello C, Sheppard V, Jay MS, Human Growth Hormone: a new substance of abuse among adolescents? Annual meeting of the society for adolescent medicine, Washington, DC, March 1992.
33 Yesalis CE, Barsukiewicz CK, Kopstein AN, et al., Trends in anabolic-androgenic steroid use among adolescent, Arch Pediatr Adolesc Med 1997; 151: 1197-206.
   Hewitt SM, Smith-Akin CK, Higgins MM, et al., Youth risk behavior surveillance: United States 1997, MMWR CDC Surveill Summ 1998; 47:61.
   Yesalis CE, Anabolic steroids in sport and exercise, 2nd ed. Champaign: Human Kinetics.
34 Newman S., Despite warnings, lure of steroids too strong for some young Canadians. Can Med Assoc J 1994; 151: 844-6.
   Canadian Centre for Drug-Free Sport. National School Survey on Drugs and Sports: final report. Gloucester, 1993.
   Laberge S., Thibault G., Dopage sportif: attitudes de jeunes athlètes québécois et significations dans le contexte d'une éthique postmoderne.
35 Kindlundh A, et al., Factors associated with adolescent use of doping agents: anabolic-androgenic steroids, Addiction (1999) 94 (4), 543-553.
   Nilsson S, Androgenic Anabolic steroid use among male adolescent in Falkenberg, Eur J Clin Pharmacol 1995; 48 (1): 9-11.
36 Lambert MI, Titlestad SD, Schwellnus MP, Prevalence of androgenic-anabolic steroid use in adolescent in two regions of South Africa, S Afr Med J 1998 Jul; 88 (7): 876-80.
   Schwellnus MP, Lambert MI, Todd M, Androgenic anabolic steroid use in matric pupils, S Afr Med J 1992; 82: 154-8.
37 Killip SM, Stennet RG, Use of performance enhancing substances by london secondary school students. London: Board education for the city of London, 1990.
38 Handelsman DJ, Gupta L, Prevalence and risk factors for anabolic-androgenic steroid abuse in Australian high school students, Int J Androl 1997; 20: 159-64.
39 ANSA: 10-11-2003.

40 Limiti F., Diffusione del doping, della creatina e degli aminoacidi tra gli adolescenti, Università La Sapienza, Roma, 2002.

41 Comune di Roma, Dipartimento Cultura-Sport, Campagna di informazione e sensibilizzazione sul problema del doping, 2003.

42 Indictment for illegal trade of hormones and substances having an anabolic effect destined to doping procedures in humans. Bologna, 21-06-2000.

43 Le Monde 13-11-2003. The Guardian 14-11-2003.

44 Indictment for illegal trade of hormones and substances having an anabolic effect destined to doping procedures in humans. Bologna, 21-06-2000.

45 Franke WW, Berendonk B, Hormonal doping and androgenization of athletes: a secret program of the German Democratic Republic government, Clinical Chemistry 43:7, 1262-1279 (1997).

46 Pattono A., Samaranch in testa all'ultima gara, Swissmoney, settembre 2000, 175-181.

APPENDIX A

Piacenza, October 1997

Four persons under arrest, 54 under criminal investigation, and 21 search warrants are the result of a police enquiry into the circulation of anabolic hormones in the commercial gymnasiums of northern Italy. Colonel Travaglione, of the Carabinieri in Rome, declares: "The scope of the illegal traffic is increasing; in 1994, 2.500 doses of anabolic hormones were seized, while in 1996 the figure rose to 176.000. This racket often uses the distributive chain used for illicit drugs."[1]

Milano, January 1999

The Carabinieri finds two bags lying on the street that contain 35 kg of testosterone. This quantity is sufficient to dope 700.000 athletes for one day or 70.000 for 10 days[2].

Torino, January 1999

The Attorney's Office of Torino opens an enquiry into expenses illegally ascribed to the Public Health Department of the Province of Torino, where in the first eight months of 1997 9 million euro were spent for EPO alone. The Health Department states that at least half of the EPO and GH that is produced and put on the market disappears on the black market that serves the sports world[3].

Sydney, January 1999

From mid-June 1997 to mid-June 1998 the Australian customs police intercepted 571 deliveries of doping substances via the Internet, mainly anabolic steroids. This trend increases as the Olympic Games approach and involves a number of countries that are building up the supplies that their athletes will use during the Games[4].

Nicosia, July 1999

Over 4.000.000 phials of erythropoietin are stolen on Cyprus. The local authorities believe that the theft was commissioned and that the product will also be distributed in the black market that supplies athletes[5].

Venice, February 2000

Thirty kilos of doping substances, produced in Greece, are seized by the Financial Police in Venice; they are mostly phials and pills of anabolic steroids contained in boxes hidden in the false bottom of a truck transporting candied fruit to Holland and Germany. The police notified investigators of the other European countries[6].

Milan, May 2000

Three persons are arrested, two Italians and an Englishman, accused of peddling drugs and doping substances (including erythropoietin); they are found to be important figures in the criminal organizations operating in Lombardy[7].

Malaga, June 2000

Torremolinos Cecil Russel, coach of the élite swimmer Nina Jivanevskaja, is arrested together with three other persons and accused of drug peddling[8].

Palermo, July 2000

After many months of investigation the Financial Police discover a widespread racket, involving a number of Italian regions, supplying erythropoietin, growth hormone and anabolic steroids for veterinary use[9].

Carrara, July 2000

Two police officers and a male nurse employed by the hospital in Carrara are arrested by the National Anti-Mafia Directorate and are accused of "involvement in the sale of erythropoietin and other drugs to professional and amateur athletes without a prescription."[10]

Sydney, July 2000

About 1000 phials containing erythopoietin are stolen from the hospital in Alice Springs; the commercial value, on the black market, amounts to several million dollars; according to the police "the phials were probably sent to Sydney."[11]

Rome, October 2000

A gigantic fraud against the National Health Service amounting to several billion Italian lire is discovered; it involves false prescriptions for anabolic steroids, erythropoietin and growth hormone[12].

Bologna, December 2000

The Attorney General concludes a widespread investigation, covering all of Italy, of the illicit traffic in doping substances; 200 search warrants are executed; 41 persons are arrested and an enormous quantity of doping substances is seized. Several European and non-European countries are involved[13].

Rome, February 2001

The UN's International Narcotics Control Council observes that during the year 2000 there has been an excessive use of drugs under medical prescription. The Report mentions "a medicalisation of social issues" and indicates that, especially in the USA, there has been a great increase in the prescription of psychoactive drugs for children under the age of six years[14].

March 2001

Two hundred thousand customers of German gymnasiums and fitness centres make habitual use of anabolic steroids. This is the result of a survey carried out by the Department of Medicine of the University of Lübeck and presented to the sports commission of the Bundestag[15].

Naples, May 2001

81 warrants are issued in 10 Italian provinces for criminal association, receiving stolen goods, corruption and fraud against the National Health Service for the recycling of stolen drugs. A police officer is among the persons arrested and is accused of buying anabolic steroids from the criminal organization and then selling them to athletes and gymnasiums[16].

Naples, July 2001

A colonel and two petty officers of the Carabinieri are arrested together along with more than ten members of criminal organizations and are accused of cigarette smuggling and peddling anabolic steroids. The Attorney's Office mentions "a rogue intelligence service capable of interfering with the regular democratic life of the country" and parallel investigations involving keeping files on members of the country's institutions[17].

July 2001

The French magazine *Santé et Travail* publishes the results of a broad survey showing that 20% of the workers use amphetamines in order to counter the effects of daily stress, while the use of cocaine is increasing among executives and managers[18].

Torino, August 2001

The Attorney's Office in Torino opens an investigation of 72 companies producing dietary supplements that contain substances having a doping effect. The FBI has identified about 10 Italian pharmacists among the buyers[19].

Torino, November 2001

An epidemiological survey carried out by the Attorney's Office in Torino on a sample of about 6.000 cyclists active between 1975 and 1995 shows over 100 cases of death caused by lymphocytic sarcoma. The number of deaths caused by melanoma and liver cancer are also above average[20].

January 2002

Phoenix police authorities in Arizona suspect there is a direct connection between a large shipment of growth hormone – 6.000 phials of Saizen worth various million dollars – and the Winter Olympics in Salt Lake City that will begin in February. Criminal organizations are involved and a police informer is killed while he is speaking over the telephone to a police officer[21].

Vienna, January 2002

On January 26, 2002, in Vienna, customs officials discover a gang of smugglers (including two police officers) preparing to sell three tons of steroids. In two warehouses, in Vienna and Tulin, the smugglers were hoarding one million seven hundred thousand anabolic tablets manufactured in the Czech Republic, having a value of one million three hundred thousand euros, and destined for sale mainly in Holland, Italy, Sweden and Spain[22].

April 2002

The IOC publishes the results of tests carried out on 634 non-hormonal dietary supplements; 94 (14.8%) are shown to be contaminated by anabolic steroids: 23 contain precursors of nandrolone and testosterone; 64 contain testosterone and 7 contain nandrolone[23].

Udine, April 2002

The Attorney General's office concludes an enquiry involving a large number of gymnasiums in northern Italy and discovers a racket involving the sale of anabolic steroids and growth hormone produced in several European and non-European countries. More than one hundred persons are under investigation. There is a close connection with a criminal enquiry in Bologna[24].

Rovereto, April 2002

The Carabinieri carry out investigations in 5 Italian regions involving the sale of anabolic steroids[25].

Brescia, May 2002

The Attorney's office in Brescia arrests three professional cyclists accused of peddling doping substances. Two deposits, used for storing significant amounts of anabolic steroids, growth hormone and erythropoietin, are discovered. The cyclists identify the supplier as a former Neapolitan police officer, Armando Marzano, who is already involved in another enquiry into the illegal trafficking of doping substances, as well as thefts from pharmaceutical stores and the pharmacies of various hospitals[26].

Naples, May 2002

Sixteen persons are arrested for involvement in the sale of doping substances to athletes and the customers of gymnasiums. The Neapolitan *camorra* (a criminal gang) is involved. Thirty persons are under investigation. The drugs came from burglaries and thefts in the following pharmaceutical deposits: Aprilia, Recanati, San Donato Milanese, Casalnuovo, Mugnano, Greggio, Sabaudia, Paternò, Monterotondo and Chiazzo. Five pharmacies are closed by order of the magistrates and eight pharmacists are arrested[27].

May 2002

Viviane Reding, European Commissioner for Sports, makes public the results of a survey, carried out in four European countries (Italy, Germany, Belgium and Portugal), on the use of anabolic steroids among the customers of gymnasiums. According to the European Union, 23.000 gymnasiums are attended by about 16.000.000 practitioners 4.6% of whom use doping substances[28].

Aosta, June 2002

A trial for illicit trafficking in anabolic steroids (involving the seizure of 170.000 doses) sold to sports centres and gymnasiums is concluded. Ten persons had been arrested[29].

Udine, June 2002

On June 1, 2002, the Judge for Preliminary Hearings in the city of Udine issued several orders for the preventive detention of certain individuals involved in illegal trafficking of anabolic steroids from Holland, Greece and Spain. From the Campania region in the south, the drugs ended up in Udine for sale in several sporting clubs and gymnasiums throughout northern Italy. Fifteen thousand packages of anabolic drugs having a value of about 300,000 euros were found and a police officer and a customs and revenue inspector were among those arrested[30].

Como, June 2002

On June 7, 2002, the customs and revenue inspectorate of the city of Como concluded a major operation involving the confiscation of doping and anabolic drugs: around 33,000 tablets and 11,000 phials, were sold to the public at prices ranging between 50 and 500 euros each. The drugs were confiscated in the provinces of Como and Liguria and came mostly from the Ukraine and Bulgaria[31].

Bolzano, June 2002

On June 29, 2002, in the province of Bolzano in northern Italy, the drug squad and the customs and excise inspectors made a spot check on the eve of a major competition for amateur cyclists and confiscated various drugs used for doping, such as erythropoietin, anabolic steroids, gonadotropin as well as narcotics. As a consequence of this raid, it was possible to trace an important network engaged in illegal trafficking[32].

Bolzano, July 2002

On July 15, 2002, again in Bolzano, five people were arrested during an investigation involving the searching of several gymnasiums, four in the southern Tyrol (Italy's Alto Adige province) and one in the Fano area. 12,000 packets of anabolic steroids were confiscated, having a value of around 250,000 euros. These investigations were originally carried out following the hospitalization of several body-builders. Large-scale traffic in narcotics was also uncovered during the investigation[33].

Brussels, July 2002

On July 23, 2002, in Brussels, one of the biggest European anti-drug operations was carried out leading to the confiscation of anabolic steroids destined for the international market. 550 kilos of hormones were discovered, having come from England and then being transported to Belgium for subsequent sale throughout Europe. The total value of the drugs amounted to 137.5 million euros. The Belgian police found out that, before sending this particular load of hormones to Belgium, the traffickers had already carried out eight or nine other similar operations for a total value of over one billion euros[34].

September 2002

On September 30, 2002, in Montecatini Terme during a national congress, the President of the Italian Society for Pediatric Medicine estimated that 5.7% of school-age young people had taken some sort of drugs to increase their success in sports[35].

Bologna, October 2002

On October 23, 2002, in Bologna, a preliminary hearing took place after the conclusion of an investigation carried out between 1999 and 2000 by the Public Prosecutor's office with the help of the Carabinieri's narcotics squad, covering over 100 sports centres and gymnasiums throughout Italy. The overall commercial value of the traffic was estimated at around 5 million euros. 75 people were arrested and charged, including several gymnasium owners and nurses. The regions involved in the investigations were Emilia Romagna, Lombardy, Veneto, Marche, Tuscany, Lazio, Campania, Sicity and Puglia. The drugs came from 10 European and non-European countries. Seventeen discotheque bouncers were also found to be implicated in the trafficking[36].

Pescara, October 2002

On October 24, 2002, in Pescara, the narcotics squad of the Carabinieri arrested the owner of a gymnasium for receiving 535 packets of doping drugs, almost all of them from abroad[37].

November 2002

On November 22, 2002, the news arrived from the United States that almost half a million young Americans use steroid drugs every year to realize their dreams of having a perfect physique. Although teenagers are the principal protagonists in this "fad", children as young as ten years old have been caught taking anabolic drugs. Border guards and customs officials are confiscating steroids from students' cars with growing frequency, the young people driving to Mexico to buy wholesale quantities of the drugs for resale at a large profit to their schoolmates. Consumption of steroids by American teenagers between 12 and 17 years old has increased by 25% in the last year[38].

November 2002

On November 23, 2002, in Naples during a Congress of the Association for Medicine in Sports, the President of the Italian Association of Pediatrics, Francesco Tancredi, spoke of the growing use of doping substances among young people: "Doping is spreading alarmingly, particularly among teenagers 16 to 18 years old, although certain investigations undertaken by the Ministry of Health show that amateur athletes are also involved. We doctors must also examine our consciences and make sure we don't forget that we are not doing our duty if we do not also practise preventive medicine." The President of the Association for Medicine in Sports, Mr. Russo, declared that "we have to use education in the schools to explain to children how to practise sports properly without dehumanizing them through the indiscriminate use of drugs."[39]

Turin, December 2002

On December 18, 2002, in Turin, the customs and revenue inspectors concluded a vast anti-drug operation that culminated in the discovery of a band of dealers responsible for the trafficking of huge quantities of Ecstasy and anabolic steroids[40].

Notes

1 ANSA (Italian Press Agency): 29-10-1997.
2 ANSA: 05-01-1999.
3 ANSA: 09-01-1999.
4 ANSA: 21-01-1999.
5 ANSA: 22-07-1999.
6 ANSA: 22-02-2000.
7 ANSA: 24-05-2000.
8 ANSA: 22-06-2000.
9 ANSA: 14-07-2000.
10 ANSA: 15-07-2000.
11 ANSA: 30-07-2000.
12 ANSA: 16-10-2000.
13 ANSA: 12-12-2000.
14 ANSA: 20-02-2001.
15 ANSA: 14-03-2001.
16 ANSA: 22-05-2001.
17 ANSA: 10-07-2001.
18 ANSA: 31-07-2001.
19 ANSA: 16-08-2001.
20 ANSA: 13-11-2001.
21 ANSA: 28-01-2002.
22 ANSA: 26-01-2002.
23 Institute of Biochemistry, German Sport University Cologne. Analysis of non-hormonal nutritional supplements for anabolic-androgenic steroids, 2002.
24 ANSA: 16-04-2002.
25 ANSA: 16-04-2002.
26 ANSA: 18-05-2002.
27 ANSA: 21-05-2002.
28 ANSA: 15-05-2002.
29 ANSA: 01-06-2002.
30 ANSA: 01-06-2002.
31 ANSA: 10-06-2002.
32 ANSA: 30-06-2002.
33 ANSA: 15-07-2002.
34 ANSA: 23-07-2002.
35 ANSA: 30-09-2002.
36 ANSA: 23-10-2002.
37 ANSA: 24-10-2002.
38 ANSA: 22-11-2002.
39 ANSA: 23-11-2002.
40 ANSA: 18-12-2002.

APPENDIX B

Transcripts of conversations intercepted by the Carabinieri narcotics squad during an operation carried out at the request of the Bologna Public Prosecutor's office

A client calls his dealer to order anabolic steroids and to ask his advice about the type of drug to use and the dosage required.

Client: **C**

Dealer: **D**

C: Listen… this week… I'll start on the Vis (*he means Testovis*)… How much should I use a week?

D: Eh…two.

C: Only?

D: Two boxes…four hundred milligrams.

C: Only?

D: Then take three…

C: When I took Viron (*he means Testoviron*) I used to take four a week, you know that, eh?

D: I know but how can you do it…they're so big.

C: So they are.

D: Eh…take six…otherwise you'll go crazy, they are two centilitres each, eh.

C: And on which days (*of the week*)?

D: Mondays, Wednesdays and Thursdays…

C: All right…what about W (*he means Winstrol*) …still three?

D: Yes, on the other three days. Tuesdays – Thursdays and Saturdays… You might even do… on Sundays…

The client calls the dealer because he has some doubts about the substances he has bought (anabolic steroids).

Client: **C**

Dealer: **D**

C: Hi, … listen… I wanted to tell you something.

D: Tell me.

C: It's about that diet you prepared for me…

D: Yes?

C: Well … but… it's … it's for … for horses?

D: Yes, of course, that's why it's even better than the other one.

C: How do you mean "better"… Hello?… Hello?

D: The composition is the same but the stuff is better… I know, I know, don't worry.

C: Are you sure?

D: Absolutely sure… Don't worry. The phials are better than the other ones.

C: … Bye bye, my girlfriend is coming.

A man, a boxing coach, who uses and peddles anabolic steroids and drugs, calls the dealer.
  Client-dealer: **CD**
  Dealer: **D**

  CD: Listen, I need a kilo of Pro (*he means Procaine, a substance notoriously used to "cut" cocaine*).
  D: Give me two days, you know whom I have to contact.
  CD: Get me also 40 boxes of Saizen.
  D: I'll give you a good price.

A dealer calls his supplier and orders hormones for an athlete who is preparing for a very important competition.
  Dealer: **D**
  Wholesale dealer: **WD**

  D: I urgently need 40 GH phials.
  WD: Which do you want?
  D: I need good stuff for someone who is preparing for the Olympic Games…
  WD: Then Humatrope is better.
  D: He needs to get stronger but without becoming bigger.
  WD: I understand, is it the same athlete who took EPO?
  D: No… I mean… but now he also needs GH.

This telephone conversation between the dealer and the wholesale dealer shows that these people have an extremely superficial knowledge as to the real content and effects of the substances they are dealing with.
  Dealer: **D**
  Wholesale dealer: **WD**

  D: What about Sustanon, you have that?
  WD: Yes.
  D: Then send me…the Polish one… what's the dosage 5 mg?
  WD: Yes… Yes… otherwise I have the Egyptian one…
  D: Egyptian, eh? What's it like?
  WD: Good… with the label… it has the right label.
  D: It has Sustanon written on it?
  WD: Yes,… it's really original.
  D: I understand… it's good then…?
  WD: Sure, sure it's good… absolutely sure it's just arrived.
  D: Ok. … send me … forty… and a hundred of… Efridene.
  WD: Um I didn't catch that.
  D: Efridene … What's the name?
  WD: Ephedrine.
  D: Ah Ephedrine sorry… Ephedrine.
  WD: Uh … What dosage? … 100?
  D: It's too strong do you think?

WD: It's meant for training?

D: Yes but… here… event the bouncers at the discos take it.

WD: Then 200 would be better… They'll feel it more.

D: You place it under the tongue, right?

WD: No. No… You just take the capsule… and swallow it… in ten minutes you…get like a punch…careful they don't kill someone.

A dealer calls a wholesale dealer because one of his clients is afraid that in the phials of anabolic steroids he bought (Winstrol) the active ingredient is missing; the wholesale dealer reassures him, saying that the laboratory where the phials were produced (obviously not the pharmaceutical company named on the label) is quite reliable and adds that, at the most, there may be a mistake on the label.

Dealer: **D**

Wholesale dealer: **WD**

Client: **C**

D: The client was told that it's just water…

WD: It's not true.

D: Why don't you talk to him and explain?

WD: All right.

C: Hello.

WD: Listen… don't worry if you can have the Phials tested.

C: Uh.

WD: Eh… They're bound to find… I'm more than sure, because I know the guy, I know he does good work.

C: Uh.

WD: Maybe, you know… when they wrote the label… maybe it didn't come out perfectly, but you can be sure that what's written is there. We're all on the same side so I would be doing harm to myself too, don't worry.

The client (a police officer) calls the dealer from the barracks, where he is on duty, to order a number of boxes of anabolic steroids for his personal use.

Client: **C**

Dealer: **D**

C: Hi. I'm…

D: Hi.

C: Where are you, at the gym?

D: No, I'm walking around.

C: Do you have the stuff with you?

D: Depends how much.

C: Can you bring me four "Oxandrolone"… 2 "Testoviron"… 2 "Proviron" in pills?

D: Four plus two plus two.

C: Hey, look, I'm on duty, I can't get out…Today I'm the officer in command…Please do me a favour…as soon as you finish at the gym…come to the gate of the barracks with the stuff.

D: Ok, bye.

The dealer calls the wholesale dealer, in front of one of his clients, to order some doping substances and ask him how to use them.

Dealer: **D**

Wholesale dealer: **WD**

D: You have to replace the boxes of RWR drive that have expired.

WD: I cant't, who will I sell them to?

D: And what do I do?

WD: Well, replace them with an equivalent substance…

D: No, they must use that one.

WD: I'm telling you it cannot be found.

D: What could I use instead?

WD: Boldone, consider that drive is Boldone plus Methandrostenolone… If you make a mixture…What are your clients like, big, thin? What do they want, more muscle or better designed muscles?

D: (talks to a man next to him) What do you want to pull or to get bigger? (then back to the wholesale dealer) He says he wants to get bigger.

WD: Then I'll give him something absolutely original, beautiful, that nobody has: Laurabolin.

D: Laurabolin…What's that?

WD: It's…for veterinary use…nobody has it, I found it in Switzerland, absolutely original.

A client calls the dealer to order anabolic steroids and ask him how to use them.

Client: **C**

Dealer: **D**

C: Listen…Can you find some equipose?

D: Yes.

C: Is it very toxic, will I tolerate it?

D: Nooo…it's like Boldone,…in fact better.

C: Like Boldone…so how many milligrams are there in a bottle?

D: Five hundred.

C: Five hundred…and how many a week?

D: Seventy-eighty, but you can go up to two hundred, it's even better.…

A client calls the dealer and tells him he will go to see him to buy some drugs. The client is preparing himself for a competition, probably body-building.

Client: **C**

Dealer: **D**

C: Hi, I wanted to ask can I come to see you on Monday?

D: Monday morning, call me and we'll agree.

C: Keep everything ready, even more than what I asked for, so we'll be ready for the competition.

D: Sure, sure.

C: You'll see I'm fantastic, you'll see I'm great.

D: Eh.

C: I'm up to a hundred kilos now, but…legs open, veins out, real great.

D: Eh.

C: But really, really great. When you'll see me you'll say "Hey, three months from the competition you're really great."

D: Well done.

C: Even the morale, everything, the diet. I feel real good, I'm following the diet you suggested, I had increased it a bit but, you know, …I'm much larger…I need another big bottle.

A dealer who is also addicted to anabolic steroids and other hormones calls his supplier to order some products and tells him of his sexual problems: from the dialogue we assume he is impotent. It's summer and the supplier is on holiday in Sardinia.

Client-dealer: **CD**

Dealer: **D**

D: I was expecting you two three days ago but you didn't show up.

CD: I couldn't make it…I was down in the dumps…

D: Why?… Did you work too much?

CD: That's right.… Then I went to bed… trouble in bed… I'm no more than "hand baggage."

D: Well, then…look I'll be back on the 31…if you need anything…

CD: Yes.

D: Let me know…I'll see what I can do.

CD: Uhm… I need some Halotestin and make sure you find what I need for my dead goose (he's referring to the fact that he's impotent). Last night it happened again, I was so ashamed, I did the best I could.

D: I haven't found any, I can't find it.

CD: Damn, I wanted to do something tonight…

D: Eh…. Too bad.

CD: When you find some Viagra keep some for me.

A few weeks later, the client calls the supplier again; the latter is back from his holiday.

Client-Dealer: **CD**

Dealer: **D**

CD: Listen, will you be in your new gym tonight?

D: Yes, from six to seven, what do you want.

CD: Ten Primo (*he means Primobolan*), Six Ox (*Oxandrolone*), then one Anapolon, and then I also need som Professor (*Profasi*)…Which do you have? 5000? Then I need…some Testo Enant (testosterone enanthate) …the one you gave me last time.

D: It's gone…I'll have it…in two or three days. I have som Sustanon.

CD: Yes… Sustanon… will be all right…give me three, then I need one multidose Winstrol…if you find any…Viagra take it, because I've gone to pieces *(he laughs)*.

D: You need it?

CD: I do, quite.

D: All right…a whole bottle…100 *(he laughs)*.

CD: Well done…it's better…about Finaject we still have some don't we? Because it's not only for me but also for other clients…

D: It will arrive you'll see.

A husband and wife work together as managers of a gymnasium and are heavily involved in peddling doping substances that they supply both to the clients of their gym and to individual amateur athletes. The husband is himself a body builder and dedicates a few hours every day to his own training. The wife is annoyed with him about this "waste of time" and every day she urges him to approach new customers and persuade them to use doping substances, especially the younger and less experienced ones.

Wife: "…That young guy who came in last night, as soon as he is ready, make sure he starts on the products."

A few days later, during another telephone conversation, she says:
"You spend more time on the athletic preparation of our customers, that's how you'll persuade them… in the meantime sell something to the one you've been working with the last few days."

A few days later she says to him:
"There are two training and integration programmes you have to get ready for, don't forget. Don't waste too much time on these deliveries, don't stop for a chat as you always do.

Her attitude changes completely when her husband is stopped by the Carabinieri, who seize a lot of GH phials and report him to the judicial authority.
Wife: **W**
Husband: **H**

W: Hello?
H: Where are you, baby?
W: Are there any problems, your voice is peculiar.
H: Ah, I was with the Carabinieri, my love.
W: Why?
H: Because they stopped me and they found…
W: Wait a minute… (*you can hear her move around swearing*)… well?
H: They found them (*the doping substances*)
W: You'll give me a heart attack…
H: But I said the substances were for my own use…
W: Idiot. All that stuff for you alone?
H: I said I had a three months preparation programme and that I take one a day.
W: Eh… shut up will you.
H: Um, I'm going home, love, to get a drink, I'm dying of thirst.
W: These things… they take years off my life.
H: All right… I'm going for a drink now.
W: You can be proud of what you've done.
H: But I'll say, listen I went to the fitness fair… I was offered the stuff… at a good price… I needed a preparation programme for myself…
W: So, you'll be known as one who takes GH.
H: Ah oh… what can I do? All right I'll go home for a drink… We'll talk later, bye now baby.
W: Bye my foot, bye.

During an enquiry the Carabinieri arrest the wholesale dealer so the dealer doesn't know where to get his supplies, so he calls the partner for news and refers to the wholesale dealer as "a soccer player."

Dealer: **D**

Wholesale dealer: **WD**

D: Listen, that guy who "used to play soccer" the one who was called "Beppe",…I haven't seen him lately…..

WD: Yes, I know.

D: He's stopped playing?

WD: Eh..I know, I know…

D: I believe he broke his leg…

WD: Eh… Eh… Eh…

D: He won't play for some time?

WD: I think he's "been put on the bench"…the doctor said he's not too well…..

D: Because we have a "match on Saturday" …I don't know what to do.… Maybe you have a suggestion?

WD: Tell me…what do you need?…

D: It'll take ten minutes "to give you the complete list".. Come to see me, I'll have it "all written down" don't forget "I'm on foot". (*he's finished all his supplies*).

WD: Eh, I know.

The dealer calls the wholesale dealer and asks for a number of products including Kriptocur (human gonadorelin) that the cyclists inhale on their way to the anti-doping laboratory in order to increase endogenous testosterone production so they can show that their testosterone level is naturally higher than normal. The other drugs as well are typically used by cyclists.

Dealer: **D**

Wholesale dealer: **WD**

D: Do you have any Testoviron?

WD: Yes.

D: How much are you asking for it?

WD: 13.000 lire a box, as usual.

D: Do you have any Kriptocur?

WD: I have two dispensers of 200.

D: How much for EPO two thousand?

WD: Sixty thousand lire.

D: And for GH?

WD: I have the 24 units one, depends on how much you need. It will cost you 360.000 lire or 330.000.

D: I want fifty phials.

WD: It's 360.000 then.

The Italian national flyweight body-building champion is one of the dealers. He works as a coach in a number of gymnasiums and supplies many practitioners with doping substances he gets from another dealer. On October 31, 1997, he was hospitalised for "acute hepatic and renal failure and rhabdomyolysis caused by diuretics abuse." He offers advice about anabolic steroids on his web site and via e-mail. He was accused of having provided the substances that caused the death of a young man on April 6, 1997.

A significant case is that of a 26-year-old customer of a gymnasium and his mother, both body builders, and both regular users of various types of hormones and other stimulating substances: Proviron, Efedrina, Moduretic, Novaldes, Clembuterolo, Decadurabolin, Testovis and Profasi.

A client who has bought a number of boxes of anabolic steroids as well as amphetamine pills calls the dealer and asks for advice.

Client: **C**

Dealer: **D**

C: Those really small pills that you told me to take when I eat…what little I do eat…what are they for?

D: To cut your appetite.

C: The small pills in the bottle?

D: Yes, in fact no…I'm making a mistake…they're to burn what you've eaten.

C: Ah. All right, because you know, I ate a sandwich a while ago…

D: A sandwich, you must be joking.

C: That's all I ate during the whole day…and I don't feel so well…

D: Stop crying all the time.

The dealer is a Municipal Councillor of a large town in the north of Italy. He calls the wholesale dealer to order various types of hormones, some of which he will sell to others while using the rest to prepare himself for a body-building competition.

Dealer: **D**

Wholesale dealer: **WD**

D: All right, I need 260 boxes of Saizen…for next week.

WD: All right, all right, I'll let you know.

D: I was expecting you the other day, you were supposed to come to see me at the town hall.

WD: Yes, I want to come to talk to you about a deal that might be interesting for both of us, I need an appointment with the mayor…

D: Do you have all my phone numbers?

WD: No.

D: Wait, I'll give them to you…Ah. I also need 300 boxes of W (WINSTROL).

A client calls the dealer to order some products and to ask his advice.

Client: **C**

Dealer: **D**

C: I called you already some time ago…I have a big problem.

D: And what is it?

C: I need to lose twenty kilos fast.

D: Why don't you exercise.

C: (*laughs*) You remember once you gave me some very good amino acids to lose weight. Can you find some for me?

D: Not today, I don't think.

C: Damn I'm desperate, I've tried everything, I'm hungry, I eat everything.

D: *laughs*.

C: I want to get back to competitions because, you remember, I had that bad accident…but I swear to you I tried, but I just can't diet. Last time I trained with those supplements and I felt good.

D: Aahh because you're a fatso (*laughs*).

C: No…I'm not…I'm not really so bad, but if I could get back to three per cent fat, like I used to be. I'm up to seventeen per cent now. I can't bear to think about it.

D: If I can find those amino acids you used to take…right now I can't remember.

C: They were the ones for cyclists remember at…

D: Well, I've written it all down.

Illegal traffic follows multiple treacherous channels, as we can see from the following dialogue between two dealers. Note that Tad 600 and Tationil are medications used for detoxication of the liver.

First dealer: **D1**

Second dealer: **D2**

D1: Do you have any Profasi?

D2: Yes.

D1: Do you also have Tad 600 and Tationil?

D2: They will find these for you.

D1: Ok. Winstrol in pills?

D2: Yes. Remember you must give me two hundred Primobolan?

D1: Yes, but don't call me at home because I've just swindled a guy and I need some fresh air.

CHAPTER 4

PROBLEMS AND PROSPECTS OF THE ANTI-DOPING CAMPAIGN

Hans B. Skaset

I would like to begin by pointing out that I am not going to approach this topic in the traditional academic manner. That does not mean that I underestimate or neglect the importance of critical academic analyses of the doping phenomenon in modern elite and mass sports. Rigorous analysis based on in-depth studies of the attitudes, behaviours and priorities of the various interest groups that belong to the national and international sports system is absolutely necessary and should be encouraged. Indeed, it is time for political scientists, sociologists, anthropologists and other qualified academics to devote more time and energy to studying the tremendous social impact of the sporting cultures of our era.

My own point of departure, however, is not an academic one. I was a national-level track and field athlete forty years ago, followed by long periods as a coach, teacher and later on as a civil servant. From the late 1960s I held fairly central positions in Norwegian sport, with continuous engagement in the anti-doping campaign at the national and international levels.

This essay offers an account of my thirty years of experience as an insider in a sports world increasingly preoccupied with maintaining its own public façade and its sense of self-importance.

National or international solutions

Before describing the main elements of the anti-doping policies I have been a part of during the last thirty years, I want to make my position on one crucial point quite clear: From the beginning of my involvement in the anti-doping campaign, I have stubbornly argued that unless there are serious national anti-doping agencies and programmes in place, the international anti-doping campaign does not stand a chance of fulfilling its mission. If national initiatives are not undertaken, or if they are postponed at the cost of unified, harmonised international solutions, the battle is doomed to fail. The administrative structure of international sports has been – and still is – so fragmented, that one cannot expect a real solution is possible at that level.

Needless to say, I fully recognise the need for international unity in the struggle against doping. Contributions to such unified international endeavours, in my view, must result from cooperation between countries. "Sport" is not something that exists outside of organised societies. Athletes are citizens of countries with cultural identities and political histories, and they do not ascend to some diffuse outer world when they move on to the level of international competition.

Sitting down and waiting for an Olympic Oracle, as most governments and national sports organisations have done for many years, has had a profoundly negative effect on the anti-doping campaign. Far too little pressure has been exerted from the national level on the international federations. The IOC and the 35 Olympic sports, that is, the international sports federations (IFs) whose sports appear in the Oplympic Programme, and most of the 30 additional so called "recognised IFs", have expressed their opinions. But they have accomplished very little in the way of developing common rules and regulations as a means of taking action against the spread of doping practises among athletes who take part in international competitions.

Passivity at the national level has contributed to allowing this laissez-faire anti-doping policy to dominate the scene over the past twenty years. One does not have to be overly suspicious to conclude that all of the parties involved – national governments, national sport organisations, international intergovernmental organisations and international sport organisations (IOC, IFs) – have allowed this situation to develop, even as they were well aware of the consequences. Anti-doping action has not been a priority, except when official declarations of this kind have seemed necessary to protect the claimed legitimacy of sport.

I would also like to point out that today, according to WADA's web site, national anti-doping agencies now exist in 22 countries. Keeping in mind that more than 200 countries are included in the more popular international sports, it is clear that vast parts of the world are not subject to any organised, reliable anti-doping activity.

I would also point out that WADA itself would not have had a chance of getting off the ground had it not been for the eight or ten fairly advanced National Anti-Doping Agencies that were already active towards the end of the 1990s. WADA's "brain trust" and operative personnel are to a large extent recruited from these national agencies. This is a tremendous paradox since the original national agencies and their activity and competence were never recognised or called on by any of the international sport bodies that "controlled" elite sport in the period leading up to the crucial period 1998-99.

National Anti-Doping Agencies: Phase One

When the anti-doping issue came to the attention of the Norwegian Confederation of Sports (NCS) in the early 1970s, it was clear from the beginning that the aim was a unified approach. All sports and all athletes organised inside the NCS were to be governed by the same rules and regulations. A centralised body, with direct access to the administrative and political leadership, had to be established. Such a body required authority and power which it could get from a unified, formalised, legal base, through the appointment of competent, sufficiently independent agency board members and through the provision of independent and stable financial resources.

The preparatory work was done at the initiative of the Executive Board of the NCS during the period 1973-75. The rules adopted by the General Assembly of the NCS in May 1976 gave the NCS the exclusive right to test all club athletes affiliated with the special sports federations of the NCS. The enforcement of sanctions was likewise reserved exclusively for the NCS.

This solution ruled out the fragmented system that would have been the result if the whole project had been dependent on whatever solution the different International Federations (IFs) might have to offer to their national affiliates. Taking into account the passive, even indifferent attitudes demonstrated by the majority of IFs, and the feeble administrative structures of national sport federations, and especially those found in the smaller and less developed countries of the world, a centralised solution created by contrast a common, unified platform for equal treatment of all Norwegian athletes, i.e. members of clubs with organised training and competition programmes affiliated with the NCS.

Fragmentation and negligence

Since 1976 I and other Norwegian anti-doping advocates have tried to get people at conferences, seminars and meetings to understand the need for unified, national solutions. Since such solutions have been seen as threats to the power of the IFs (and the IOC), which have openly argued that national affiliates and their athletes were responsible for solving their own problems, the anti-doping campaign has been effectively retarded over a period of at least twenty years. As stated above, the IFs did not support their national affiliates to the degree that would have permitted the development of national sport-specific anti-doping programmes. Most IFs, the Olympic sports included, were not empowered, equipped or willing to give the necessary priority, resources and attention to an issue that was complicated and negative in nature, and that had the potential to impair the attractiveness of their competitions. Decreased performance levels could not easily be sold in a media-driven sports world bred on record-breaking performances.

The IOC has concentrated its efforts on laboratory accreditation, the list of prohibited substances, and testing procedures during Olympic competitions. But it had, up to 1999, done nothing to promote the anti-doping campaign through the National Olympic Committees (NOCs), of which there are today 199. This network could have been a useful, and perhaps even a truly effective, world-wide system to spread the gospel of anti-doping down to the national level. As I shall later make clear, the NOCs were not engaged by the IOC in any anti-doping campaign between the Games, and for obvious reasons: The IOC did not want to take responsibility for anything but the 16 days of Winter and Summer Olympic Games. Almost all of the athletes' time in and out of training was the responsibility of the IFs, and their national affiliates. This doctrine saved the IOC from possible conflicts with the IFs that might have resulted from an intrusion on their territory. Accordingly, the IOC tried to avoid any association with unsavoury conflicts over doping which might have jeopardised the Olympic image.

As a consequence, the NOCs remained silent and passive during the entire Samaranch presidency (1980-2001). At the opening of the Olympic Congress in Baden-Baden (1981), the newly elected IOC-President proclaimed that the "Olympic Movement" stood firmly behind him, and that it would fight the evils of the "artificial athlete". Rhetoric aside, the IOC has not in fact used its own eligibility rules to bar athletes who have been banned for doping from participating in Olympic Games. The IOC has on certain occasions talked about suspending Olympic sports with evident doping problems from the Olympic programme. But this issue has never reached the top of the IOC's agenda for reasons which are obvious: The result would be open political conflict inside "the Family," and this would make a negative impression on the multinational corporations that advertise themselves at the Games.

Keeping the Games "clean" has been the stated aim of the IOC. As long as "Clean Games" meant no doping incidents during the 16 Olympic Days, this goal was in fact quite realistic, except for the problems deriving from the inclusive Olympic Family Policy. All NOCs were accorded a minimum representation paid for by the IOC. This policy represented a certain threat, however, because it gave access to the Games to certain ill-informed and marginal members of the Olympic Family. Confronted with the temptations of the professional sports world, athletes and leaders from less developed regions might be tempted to try to catch up with the lost years of preparation by doping during the 16 days of Olympic competition. What athletes did during the days, weeks and years prior to the Games was not the responsibility of the IOC. That responsibility rested firmly with the autonomous IFs, which were fierce competitors in the television and sponsor markets and relied on the IOC's support and protective actions that favoured the most devoted "family members."

National Anti-Doping Agencies: Phase Two

As doping techniques developed during the 1980s and 1990s, some countries with national agencies began a more or less formal cooperative anti-doping effort. A central feature at this stage was the involvement and engagement of national governmental agencies along with agencies belonging to the sports movements of the countries involved. On the Nordic level this cooperation developed gradually and led to closer contact between the governmental organisations and non-governmental organisations, thereby reducing the tendency to resort to turf battles when problems arose. Cooperation was, for obvious reasons, absolutely necessary. Even if it had established a centralised, competent anti-doping agency, the national sports movement could not cope with the growing problems of the illegal importation and distribution of doping substances. The need for legal support and action from government agencies became apparent. The spread of doping practices to younger athletes, and to groups outside of organised sports, required public authorities to engage in this matter, for reasons having to do with health and possible criminal activity. The growing severity of the doping problem, and its links to the much larger drug problems of entire societies, made it necessary to engage governmental agencies outside of the ministry that was traditionally responsible for sports issues.

Targeted state grants

During this second phase of development, i.e. the period from the beginning of the 1990s, the Norwegian government earmarked state grants for the activities of the centralised anti-doping agency affiliated with the sports organisations. The reason for this was that the sports organisations' decision-making body entrusted with dividing up the state funding for sports had internal problems regarding priorities. The traditional interests of sports organisations dominated the internal agenda. Anti-doping initiatives were still considered an expensive and sometimes unnecessary burden. Even after 15 years of national anti-doping activities, the leading sports officials had not become accustomed to the idea that they had to take permanent responsibility for the effects of their own pursuit of athletic excellence.

In order to circumvent this situation some governments, including the Norwegian government, started a new budgetary procedure which earmarked a portion of the state funding for anti-doping activity. This amount was set aside exclusively for anti-doping purposes and could not be reduced or diverted to other purposes by the Executive Board of the NCS. Due to this intervention by the state, the National Anti-Doping Agency was made financially secure and given the authority to operate according to its fundamental purpose.

From the very beginning the sports organisations were eager to declare that they were able to handle their doping problems without interference from state agencies. National and international sports organisations had sung this tune for years and well into the 1990s. The result, unfortunately, was that most governments, for political and opportunistic reasons, kept their distance from the anti-doping activities of the sports organisations. The overall effect was that the doping problem spread without serious resistance in most countries, both in Europe and even more so in other parts of the world. The sports movement's anti-doping strategy, along with the passive position adopted by most governments, contributed to a situation that benefited only those bent on performance enhancement, commercial exploitation, and media exposure.

A memorandum of understanding and IADA

In the early 1990s, some of the governments that were on speaking terms with their national sports organisations regarding the anti-doping issue started a dialogue with the aim of demonstrating their common purpose. These countries firmly believed that the anti-doping struggle could not succeed without strong national support for centralised, effective anti-doping agencies. These agencies had to have the support of the sports organisations as well as the governments, whether they were legally constituted independent agencies or still operating within the national sports organisations.

The Canadian government, along with their British and Australian counterparts, came up with a "Memorandum of Understanding" that outlined what governments could do to create more momentum in the anti-doping struggle and what kinds of reciprocal responsibilities the Memorandum implied. Norway subscribed to this Memorandum in 1992 after a formal meeting between the responsible ministers of Canada and Norway during the Winter Games in Albertville. Later on France and New Zealand were included in the agreement.

The Memorandum of Understanding was a useful start, even if it included a long list of formalities. Eventually, the formal platform was altered when the Memorandum period came to an end. A less formal platform was developed, called the International Anti-Doping Arrangement (IADA), which towards the end of the 1990s came to include Holland, Sweden, Denmark and Finland, as well as the original signatories, or nine countries in all. (France had in the meantime withdrawn from the agreement.) The IADA countries held two meetings each year, and also convened at the Council of Europe (Monitoring Group) and at other international conferences where doping or related issues were discussed. It was at a meeting in Oslo in 1995 that IADA countries decided to seek accreditation through the ISO (International Organisation for Standardisation) system, which meant a considerable leap forward in control standards and in operational procedures. By the end of the 1990s, the IADA countries were either in conformity with the ISO standards or were in the process of qualifying for accreditation.

The IADA countries, in my view, soon became influential players on the international scene, not because of a large number of members, but because of the serious and competent work carried out by the member countries. Forming this political alliance enabled them to show other countries how a serious contribution to the anti-doping struggle could be made.

We all knew the alternative to such an arrangement too well. The Council of Europe, for example, had the "Anti-Doping Convention" it adopted in 1989. As the chair of the Monitoring Group (i.e. the Steering Group) of this Convention for four years (1990-94), I had ample opportunity to observe the standards of knowledge and the involvement of the representatives of participating countries in meetings, seminars and working groups. This enabled me to see the difference between the proclaimed intentions of the Convention and what it actually meant to sign and then ratify. About 30 European countries signed and ratified the Convention during the first half of the 1990s, the majority of which had little or no organised, effective anti-doping activity at the national level. The Anti-Doping Convention of the Council of Europe was open to all. It was against the working principles of the Council of Europe to evaluate a country's ability or willingness to take on the obligations of the Convention before joining, or to evaluate a country's compliance with the requirements after a certain time had passed. As a consequence, the Convention's contribution to moving the anti-doping campaign forward was seriously harmed by its willingness to accept every Tom, Dick and Harry into the fold.

The IADA countries kept in close touch with each other during the Monitoring Group's meetings and tried in various ways to introduce stricter rules that could prevent countries from "hiding behind" the Anti-Doping Convention of the Council of Europe. Although a plan for voluntary evaluation of compliance with the requirements of the Convention was introduced, it did not prove to be adequate. Its voluntary basis and a lack of financial and human resources hampered effective implementation of this plan. Countries were reluctant to present themselves as candidates for inspection, and the money needed to establish and maintain evaluation teams across Europe was never included in the Council of Europe's budget.

After the 1998 scandals

I will refrain from commenting on the farcical anti-doping efforts of the Italian National Olympic Committee (CONI) or the débâcle of the 1998 Tour de France that produced a sense of crisis and undermined the credibility of the anti-doping endeavours of the IOC and the international federations (IFs). The Lausanne anti-doping conference of February 1999 was, therefore, an attempt by the IOC and the IFs to regain control over a situation that was now spinning out of their control.

For the first time, governments were invited to a meeting of this kind, and some of the government ministers in attendance expressed strong and critical opinions to the leadership of the IOC and IFs. All such criticisms were of course, taken as blatant insults by the IOC members and other international officials. The "Family" was shocked when the German Minister of the Interior, Mr. Schily, speaking on behalf of the European Union, addressed President Samaranch directly and asked him to accept the consequences of the IOC's failure and step down.

The invitation extended to the government ministers was, however, a strategic move by the IOC. After 20 years of negligence and neglect, the IOC leadership finally understood that doping in sport was a global problem that could not be handled by a fragmented international sport system alone. The IOC's invitation to the governments to take a role alongside the "Olympic Family" in the fight against doping was not made with pleasure. The IOC more than hinted that sport's doping problem was just a reflection of drug problems among modern youth everywhere, and that sport was a victim of larger problems that the politicians had not solved.

The IOC had set aside USD 25 million for the new agency that would go into operation before the end of 1999, and the governments were invited to come on board if they could come up with an equivalent amount of money. One can imagine what Dick Pound of the IOC was thinking when he challenged the representatives of the governments to respond to this invitation. It is unlikely he expected them to meet his challenge.

The ministers of the IADA countries met at the end of the conference in Lausanne for the purpose of exchanging ideas regarding the issues that had come up during the conference. I mention this in order to emphasize the importance of IADA as an instrument for building political alliances.

My personal opinion was – and still is – that governments should be very cautious and not fall into what might be seen as a trap. Collaboration with the Olympic Movement in the fight against doping could be acceptable if the authority were equally shared. But this was not the emerging picture by the end of the Lausanne meeting. My advice to the Norwegian minister was not to support direct government participation in the new agency, and not to support the new structure with government funds. Instead the governments should concentrate their efforts on developing national anti-doping agencies in as many countries as possible, through bilateral and multilateral action. The money requested by the Olympic Movement from the governments for the new world body should instead be reserved for the support of new national anti-doping agencies.

This is not the place to comment on the position of the representatives of the Council of Europe in the months after the Lausanne meeting. That also includes the leading (chair) EU country at that time. In my opinion, both institutions were quickly co-opted into the IOC's prepared agenda and were too eager to comply with the expectations of the IOC.

The Sydney Summit and the IICGADS-meetings

Even before the Lausanne meeting, the Australian Government had announced its intention to organise a meeting for some 25 selected countries before the 2000 Sydney Olympic Games. The Sydney Summit took place in November 1999. The most significant political outcome was that an international intergovernmental consultative group on anti-doping work was established at the initiative of the Canadian government. This Intergovernmental Group, which had the IADA countries at its core, held a separate meeting in Sydney and decided to meet again in Montreal in February 2000.

The two most pressing issues in Montreal were the distribution of seats between the Olympic Movement and the Governments in the new WADA structure (its Foundation Board and Executive Board), and the distribution of seats among the governments of the different regions (continents). The financial issue was to be the main item on the agenda at the Oslo meeting of IICGADS in November 2000.

As mentioned above, I headed the preparations for the Oslo meeting until October 30, 2000. On that day I resigned as Director General after not being supported by the minister of culture in a conflict with the leadership of the Norwegian Olympic Committee over Norway's position vis-à-vis the doping problem.

Final Comments

In my previous remarks I noted that over the past 25 or 30 years my own position on the doping problem has not changed. I have consistently emphasised the need for effective national solutions in the anti-doping struggle. It will be possible to keep the doping problem under some degree of control only if there is real cooperation between the sports organisations and the governments.

This position does not exclude solutions based on international cooperation. At the same time, international cooperation at this level should involve the national anti-doping agencies of various countries as well as the traditional national and international bodies.

The assumption that international athletes exist outside the jurisdiction of their native countries, that they "belong" to and are the responsibility of their international sports organisations, is both contrary to common sense and dangerously misleading. The anti-doping campaign has, in fact, been greatly hampered by the persistent influence of such notions. The passive attitudes that result from such false beliefs have resulted in lost opportunities for doping control and in too many opportunities for practitioners of doping.

The WADA structure means that governmental representatives will continuously risk being taken hostage by the Olympic Movement. The phrase "ministers come and go" is in this case all too true. If we compare the representatives on the Foundation Board of WADA in 2000 with the Board representatives of today, you find that the government list has changed considerably, while the representatives of the Olympic Movement have not changed at all. It is simply naïve to assume that this will not affect how WADA does business. The shared interests and self-protective instincts of the experienced representatives of the Olympic Movement should not be overlooked or underestimated.

A centralised body headquartered in Montreal can develop rules and regulations for 35 Olympic international federations, and even for the additional 30 federations recognised by the IOC. Beyond these 65 IFs there are still around 20 IFs in the loose GAISF (General Association of International Sports Federations) structure which will have to be attended to if the doping problem in sports is to be dealt with effectively. WADA may be able to test international athletes in and out of competition, and perform tests of up to four or five thousand athletes. This will be done, however, at great cost to the stakeholders, and it will not reach the grass roots level where young athletes are developed.

Since WADA will never be able to take responsibility for the young, aspiring athletes of the world, it will be up to national anti-doping agencies all over the world to do so. Unless these athletes are given the right kind of advice and education while their minds are still receptive, the international initiatives being promoted by the WADA leadership are likely to fall far short of their goals.

CHAPTER 5

BIOGRAPHICAL RISKS AND DOPING

Karl-Heinrich Bette

Every biography involves risks, since there is no life that can be fully planned and guided. Somehow there are always obstacles that disrupt our plans. It is no accident that many existential philosophers have pointed out that failure is to be counted among the fundamental human experiences, and that an appropriate engagement with risks, unpredictable events and the various blows of fate is what the art of survival is all about. Nor are athletic careers exempt from surprises and uncertainties. In addition to the normal problems of life in complex societies which elite athletes, like other members of society, have to master, athletes are subject to special circumstances that appear neither in other social sectors nor, to a comparable degree, in the elite sport of an earlier period. This change in the circumstances in which athletic careers are pursued is linked to the changed significance of contemporary sport. Athletic contests are exciting, they allow people to live vicariously through their emotions, and they encourage widespread hero-worship. The emotional reactions that are catalyzed in spectators at major sporting events have made elite sport more attractive to corporate interests, politicians, and the mass media. In recent years we have seen the emergence of a constant demand for high-level sports performances, with the result that the role of risk-taking in athletic careers has taken on an entirely new role.

The paper that follows will show that the spread of doping is largely a consequence of the altered circumstances in which elite athletes pursue their careers. For it has become clear that increasing numbers of athletes are engaging in deviant practices to deal with the opportunities and risks that have become a part of their lives. Indeed, they cannot help but take the physical, psychological and social risks and consequences involved. First we must describe the *typical risk-factors of athletic careers*, so that we may then analyze *doping as a coping strategy* that grows out of these specific risks. A third section presents *opportunities for anti-doping work from a sociological perspective* under the rubric of "managing risk patterns."

This should make it clear that, contrary to some familiar and premature judgments, doping is not something that can simply be traced back to the personality traits of individual athletes, coaches, officials or sports physicians. Doping is less a case of "bad" people than of social conditions that produce deviance in predictable ways. As a sociologist, one might well ask, how is it that elite sport has brought together such an assortment of actors, that irrespective of discipline or nationality, collectively demonstrate so many character flaws? The sheer number of offenses and the increasing rate of deviance should make us think more deeply about what is going on. A look at the biographical characteristics of elite athletes can teach us a great deal about the socially conditioned dimension of doping-related deviance.

Risk Factors in Athletic Careers

The major risk that is run by those involved in competitive sport as athletes is that they will not be successful during their careers. To be sure, this statement appears at first to be banal, yet it is precisely this obvious point about failure that can become a problem for the individual athlete. This lack of success can have many causes. Failure is the predictable result of elite sport's focus on competition. Sportive competitions produce losers in a systematic way so as to focus attention on the winners. Failure is, therefore, not an accident but the reality to which one must adapt. To put it more precisely, athletic competition requires lots of losers so that a few victors can distinguish themselves. The winners are thus comparable to parasites that feed on the inferior. The legitimate production of the failure of the many in favor of success for the few is a central element in the drama of athletic competitions. Although official Olympic rhetoric still proclaims that taking part is everything, the rule of every contest is that the athlete who finishes in second place is already the first among the losers.

During the 1996 Atlanta Olympic Games, the sporting goods manufacturer Nike summed this up in a concise formula: "You didn't win silver, you lost the gold." Even if the higher ranked performances can be celebrated as successes, despite this exaggerated judgment, the compassion of the crowd is extended to those who have finished in "thankless fourth place." The collective memory of elite sport preserves above all the names and performances of the victors. The losers are remembered as actors who tried but did not succeed. The cold-hearted division into ranks that results from the code of victory and defeat is particularly apparent in the care with which winners are separated from losers when the human senses can no longer make such distinctions, one example being the introduction of hundredths of a second in swimming and athletics competitions.

For the individual athlete, failures in the course of a career must be expected, and especially in those disciplines in which global competition makes the intensity of the competition particularly fierce. Indeed, for a century or more elite sport has been a global arena of self-assertion. As a matter of principle it includes everyone, since it is immune to discriminating criteria such as race, class, gender and age. Everyone who accepts the rules and produces performances that correspond to them can participate. For the lives of the athletes this principled openness has enormous consequences: Any time athletes from many countries compete against each other in hard-nosed competitions, they become real threats to each other. Elite athletic careers fail because some athletes are simply better than others. The more that elite sport takes on the status of a subsystem of global society the greater the social significance of a discipline and the more likely it is that the individual athlete will fail.

Biographical risks in elite sport do not simply result from the defeats that one has to deal with in any competition. The high degree of uncertainty that characterizes athletic careers arises on account of something that distinguishes elite sport from other social enterprises in a very particular way, namely, the *extreme dependency on the body that marks the athletic enterprise*. In the context of a normal life the body is the primary site for the satisfaction of consumer needs, whether this means sexual experience or feelings of well-being that are made possible by eating or drinking. An athlete, however, has to establish an instrumental relationship to his own body. This is a consequence of the individuality of performance and of the "technical" dependency on the body that is part of athletic success. The body-ideal of the elite athlete is the body that functions best in a specific discipline and that can be further developed in that direction. This body-image stands in stark contrast to the sensual satisfactions of everyday life. Injuries and declining performances are perceived as crises that are to be avoided, eliminated, or postponed. Because ever smaller improvements in performance can only be achieved by means of ever greater levels of exertion, the danger of overstressing the body of the athlete is an integral part of an athletic career. In the world of elite sport, career plans can be ruined overnight if the body refuses to perform.

In a society that otherwise does so much to repress the body, it is this indispensable role of the body, which makes elite sport so uncommonly interesting. Yet this is also the Achilles' heel of the entire system and of those who make a career out of elite sport. Every athlete runs the risk of failure on account of injuries, illness and declining performance. The athlete's dependence on his body introduces an uncertainty into his experience and actions that does not occur in other fields of endeavor. The status of an athlete is, for this reason, more fragile than that of an academic researcher whose credentials have nothing to do with physical competence, and who can fulfill his professional obligations in a competent manner even if physical decline has already set in. Comparable qualifications are found only in work roles based on physical performance, as in dance or in the fashion and advertising industries that are so fixated on beauty and youthfulness. Missing here, of course, is the formal competition in pursuit of an elusive victory.

Defeats in competition and the career problems that result from them are not just the result of able opponents, intensely competitive sports disciplines, and reluctant bodies. The only athletes who can make it over the long haul in elite sport are those who are psychologically robust enough to withstand the pressures of competition and success. In these circumstances, there is always the risk that, even after the years of effort that have been invested, one may *lose his motivation*. A psyche that at some point decides that enough is enough, because it has been overtaxed by anxiety, expectations of success, injuries, or its public role, can put an abrupt end to an athletic career. For that reason, athletes who are interested in maintaining their reputations have to preserve their motivation to perform for a corresponding period of time. Anyone whose motivation lags behind his performances may well wind up as a tragic hero in the annals of his sport.

Failure as the major risk of athletic careers can also originate in *the manner in which performances are measured as well as changes in context that inhere in a particular sport*. It thus makes a difference whether athletic performances, as in the case of athletics, can be objectified in terms of centimeters, grams and seconds, or whether they are defined by referees. The degree to which the nature of measurement in a particular sport can influence athletic careers is demonstrated over and over again by the controversies about points that are awarded, or by the nominations in the artistic sports such as rhythmic gymnastics, sports gymnastics, traditional gymnastics, and ice skating or in combat sports such as boxing or wrestling. The arbitrary nature of nominations to competitions and the judgments made by referees create situations in which athletes can feel abandoned and quite helpless.

Many careers have had to end without having achieved any international successes, because the nature of the sport had changed in a fundamental way. For example, federations may change how competitions are organized, they might modify weight classes or eliminate entire Olympic disciplines – all of which can disrupt the planning of a career and require a new kind of athlete. Olympic boycotts, too, as in Moscow (1980) and Los Angeles (1984), are events to which no athletic career can adjust. Many athletes have had to give up their medal hopes overnight, because politicians had made sport into an instrument for their own purposes.

Risks to athletic careers can also result from *the scarcity and instability of favorable conditions* for athletic development. An athlete who finds himself at a particular stage of his career and who is not willing or able to adapt to institutional requirements, will have a very hard time winning competitive opportunities even as a latecomer or as someone entering from another discipline. In a social enterprise which distributes its resources according to the law of Matthew ("To those who have will be given; from those who have not will be taken"), missing out on institutionally sponsored training will sooner or later mean leaving the discipline. Top performances without the benefits of a supportive training milieu are very unlikely. For no athlete can meet the requirements of modern elite sport, simply on the basis of his own resources. Without a coach, sports physician or physiotherapist, and without the corresponding training opportunities and logistical support, many recent performances could not have been achieved. If training conditions are interrupted, because the family, the sports association or sponsors are not there to offer their support, or if state funding disappears, or if certain disciplines decline in popularity, then one can predict that some careers will come to an end. And if losses lead to a withdrawal of resources and then further losses, the result is a cycle of failure that ends in no support at all. And so it becomes clear that elite athletic careers are vulnerable, not only to the standard competitive situation that involves winning and losing, but also to a second aspect of competition, namely, the struggle for scarce opportunities to obtain support and the chance to enter competitions. Losing in this competition is a very risky business.

Yet another risk factor for athletic careers results from *the actual or presumed incidence of doping in a particular discipline, as well as the reluctant and procrastinating attitudes of many sports federations in the area of anti-doping initiatives.* The fact that suspicions about, and not necessarily the reality of, doping present a serious risk to athletic careers has to do with the fact that doping can literally come out of nowhere as a self-fulfilling prophecy. The athletes need only *think* that their opponents are doping to have a rational reason to dope themselves. Unproven doping insinuations can quickly lead to a situation in which doping becomes a hedge against incurring a disadvantage. And this predicament applies to national federations as well as to athletes. These reciprocal entanglements have consequences for athletic careers. Federations which do not take their doping control obligation seriously, so as to remain internationally competitive, put pressure on their athletes to dope without intending to do so, thereby becoming a part of the problem they claim to be solving. This means that *the widespread aversion to risk of many sports federations in the anti-doping campaign presents a grave risk to athletic careers,* since half-hearted doping control, or no doping control at all, makes it necessary for athletes to engage in deviant practices in order to adapt to the doping of other athletes.

The risk factors described so far can, last but not least, produce cumulative effects and create many causal interdependencies. For example, athletes who want to minimize the risk of losing by intensifying their training regimens will eventually exert stress on their minds and bodies in such a way as to lead to injuries and diminished motivation. It can also happen that athletes who dope themselves in doping-dependent disciplines, in pursuit of scarce training resources and competitive opportunities, run the risk of exposure and social stigmatization.

A further intensification of this already volatile situation arises in that lack of success presents a threat, not just to the individual athlete, but to everyone involved in producing performances. Coaches, officials, clubs and federations, corporate and political sponsors all have a stake in success. It is precisely those people who are professionally employed in elite sport and have no career alternatives who are under pressure to make sure that the athlete they either take care of or sponsor is successful no matter what. The coach's position and career are on the line; sports physicians are judged, not on whether they promote health, but on whether they have the athlete ready for competitions. For clubs and federations, state funding, payments from sponsors and perhaps television revenues are all at stake. And the sponsors need a continuous series of successes, because otherwise the public and potential advertisers will lose interest.

Failures, therefore, affect not only individual athletes but are also events that affect the athlete's support system both inside and outside the environment in which he trains. This creates *a dangerous reduplication and intensification of the risk level,* in that there is a *heightening of risk on account of exaggerated demands* on the athlete. Everything having to do with relaxation, innocence, and spontaneity is driven out of sport and replaced by calculation and demands based on what is expected of the athlete. The athletes wind up in a situation which further accentuates the high-cost status of what they do.

Quite apart from the risks associated with failure, athletes' lives are vulnerable to a second type of risk regarding *uncertainty about the future after the end of an athletic career*. The future only becomes an issue when one's own performances stagnate or decline, injuries occur, or one confronts outside factors that can restrict an athletic career. Even if athletes escape such disruptions, they can still anticipate such things happening in their own lives.

An initial risk factor results from *closure of the athlete's ability to think and make judgments*. Athletes who define their identity primarily through athletic success, and are confirmed in this identity by their competitive community, run the risk of losing both their sense of meaning and identity after the end of an athletic career. When the physical and mental ability to compete declines, and the cycle of defeat has become irreversible or is about to set in, many athletes experience the traumatic moment of stopping and saying goodbye to a self-image that has been determined by years of almost exclusive fixation on elite sport. This produces the feelings of emptiness that affect both male and female athletes after their careers are over.

Many athletes speak of falling into a deep hole. Those who have spent much of their lives integrated into sports communities experience withdrawal symptoms when they have to give up this "social uterus." The risk is in losing sport as a safe haven and in experiencing a "social death" (Rosenberg 1984), in that they must give up the power, income, and social opportunities that come with the life of an athlete. Anyone who has not pursued educational or professional alternatives, or who has neglected to win or to convert athletic laurels into other "currencies," will find the end of a career especially painful. Additional uncertainties result from the economic risk involved in having invested years in elite sport which may have resulted in physical injuries.

Coping by Doping: Themes

Deviant behavior that takes the form of secret doping does not, as the previous analysis should have made clear, simply come out of nowhere. As the American sociologist of technology Charles Perrow (1984) has put it, doping is much better described as a "normal accident" which constantly assumes new forms that arise from evolving social conditions. In an abstract sense doping points to the escalating logic of elite sport itself (citius, altius, fortius) and the way it is unleashed in competition. To the extent that big money, television ratings, and political interests come into play, the pressure for success exerts increasing pressure on everyone involved. Between the athlete and the public there is a complex relationship which articulates expectations about success and goes so far as to give this relationship a contractual aspect.

These structural changes and their inflationary demands threaten to overwhelm athletic careers. The internal control mechanisms that competitive sport has developed, such as Fair Play initiatives and sports ethics, are now under enormous pressure.

Legitimate innovations such as technique, tactics and training are losing their role as the primary motor of progress that drives athletic performances. As unwanted as they are inevitable, probing and experimenting in the borderline and forbidden zones of performance-enhancement are now a part of elite sport. Seen against this background, doping appears, not as an accidental aggregation of individual cases, but rather as a coping strategy which many athletes use in an attempt to counteract the risks they run. *Intentional doping in elite sport serves as a kind of multi-purpose weapon to prevent failure and to minimize the uncertainty about the future that comes in the wake of an athletic career.*

The following general themes are, therefore, useful for theorizing about the situation in which elite athletes find themselves:

Athletes dope primarily *to avoid failure in athletic competitions.* The uncertainty about who wins and who loses is supposed to be transformed into a certainty about one's own chances. In this sense, doping aims at disabling central aspects of the success principle that lies at the heart of sport, namely, the principle of open competition and the idea of the participants' formal equality.

Athletes also use doping as a strategy *to boost the body's physical capacities and to neutralize its limitations.* Targeted interventions are supposed to adapt the fallible athletic body to the demands of the various sports disciplines. Athletes, coaches, and support personnel strive to devise a program that will optimize the cause-effect relationship between what is invested and the goal at which everyone is aiming. The use of EPO, anabolic steroids and other drugs and procedures aims at achieving a precisely specified output in a reliable manner.

Our third point is that, for a growing number of athletes, *doping has clearly become the procedure of choice for adjusting the mind to the demands of elite sport.* Doping is used, for example, to eliminate the adverse effects of anxiety or excitement, to solve motivation problems, or to produce calm or relaxation in competitive situations. One intervenes in the body in order to prepare the mind for competition and success.

Fourth, doping comes into play *when athletes want to eliminate the risk of missing out on scarce institutional resources.* Participation in the various competitions sponsored by clubs, federations, and other sponsoring organizations is, in the last analysis, an indispensable prerequisite for staying at the elite level. Competitive failure involves the risk of not having access to these resources or of being cut off from them altogether. Athletes thus weigh the possibilities and make rational choices about whether the risk of losing resources is greater or smaller than the risk of being caught. The fact that we are seeing more and more strategies involving illegitimate innovations, in addition to the many opportunities offered by legitimate innovations, tells us something about the directions in which these calculations are headed.

Fifth, doping responds to *the implicit pressure to dope as well as to the tacit acceptance of doping in many federations.* Athletic careers are put at risk when federations behave passively toward doping. Doping thus appears as an epiphenomenon resulting from un-solved doping control problems at the federation level. The fact that, in most disciplines, doping is a defensive rather than an offensive strategy shows that the federations make their own contribution to doping by implementing deficient doping control measures. Athletes who are making up their minds whether or not to dope will sometimes get clear signals from the federations that borderline doping is valued more highly than adherence to rules about fairness.

Sixth, doping can be a *strategy for asserting one's identity*. The performance-oriented individualism of today's elite athlete takes the code of victory at its word and creates a kind of identity that athletes neither can nor want to give up. The only chance for distinguishing oneself consists in being better than the others. In this context, pills and injections provide the self-image of the athlete with successful experiences and ward off the threats to this identity that come from failure.

Seventh, doping is *a way of reducing economic risks*. Scientific technologies are supposed to produce a more reliable return on one's investment. For without competitive successes there will be no funding from sports organizations or from sponsors. This creates a pressure on the athlete due to high expectations, even as an athletic career of limited duration must demonstrate success – and this in a situation where all the other competitors are striving toward the same goals.

Eighth, doping can take the form of *secondary deviance*. Doping deviance must be kept secret if performances that have been achieved by means of doping are not going to be denounced as doping records after the fact. Doping deviance thus leads to other forms of deviance, and so on. And it becomes difficult to extricate oneself from this cycle.

The most difficult aspect of this situation consists in the fact that doping is an *overdetermined phenomenon*. Any one of the motives mentioned so far will suffice to cause athletes to dope themselves or be doped by others. This makes the campaign against doping unusually difficult and has persuaded not a few opponents of doping that this campaign is, in fact, a hopeless enterprise. Even if one motive for doping has been brought more or less under control – such as providing professional opportunities that will be available after the athletic career is over – there are many other factors that can induce athletes to dope: doping to assert one's identity, to avoid competitive disadvantages and failures, to take advantage of economic opportunities, or to compensate for injuries or age-related performance declines.

The fact that these risk patterns exist does not mean that the risk elements involved in planning an athlete's career are determined in advance. The relationship between context and action is better understood as a nonlinear connection. For how else could one explain as a sociologist that many athletes who operate in the same or a similar context do *not* dope? Intervening variables which substitute for ethical motives and prevent doping include: exceptional talent, the fear of being found out, the stigma attached to addiction and illness, the moral support of a family or club, a lack of money, or lack of access to a deviant subculture.

Athletes thus have opportunities for shaping their own lives which they will make use of with varying degrees of skill. The risk factors we have discussed must be understood

KARL-HEINRICH BETTE

as factors which direct or otherwise affect the athlete's behavior. The athlete's own actions cannot, however, significantly influence, let alone abolish, the general attitude toward competition, the dependency on the body, or the degree to which a specific discipline is affected by doping. And anyone who develops an antipathy toward the merciless logic of victory and defeat or his discipline's way of judging performance would be better off getting out of elite sport.

The high frequency of scandals shows that, despite opportunities not to do so, many athletes look upon doping as a rational choice of action, apart from those cases in which athletes are doped without their knowledge by coaches, doctors or competitors. Still, doping as a career strategy plays a highly ambivalent role. While it is intended to reduce uncertainties, it produces instead no more than a false security, because it is extremely risky. Even short-term gains achieved through the use of new drugs or procedures come, as we know, at the price of serious physical and psychological consequences – not to mention the risk of being caught and suffering a "social death" as in the case of Ben Johnson.

In addition, the secrecy that isolates competitors from each other leads to an intensifying spiral into deviance. Global competition thus threatens to turn into a "race between fools" (Hirsch 1980: 96) in which all of the participants must bear the negative consequences of this sort of behavior.

Anti-Doping Work as a Management Problem

Given the multifactorial basis of the motivation to dope, and the compatibility of deviance and the logic of elite sport, it is clear that we are still far from having a solution to the doping problem. Doping cannot be totally eliminated precisely because it is so closely bound up with the risks of an athletic career and the dilemmas faced by sports federations. A radical solution of the doping problem is thus not feasible, because elite sport is embedded in a stable social configuration (see Bette/Schimank 1995, 1996, 2000) whose major actors come from the economic sector, political life, the mass media and the general public. All we can reasonably expect is to confine doping within certain limits.

The anti-doping measures that have been undertaken to date fall into two general categories: controls and penalties on the one hand, and educational efforts on the other. Doping controls are retroactive in nature, and they have had little success up to this point. But even if control measures could be considerably improved, there remains the problem that they do not prevent doping but only deal with an act of deviance that has already occurred. Over time the penalties may produce a deterrent effect, although this requires a heavy and continual investment in the control effort.

In contrast to penalties, which should be regarded as external strategies, educational efforts aim at establishing a sense of values inside athletes themselves. This means that the athlete himself is in a position to reject the temptations that arise. Fair Play and ethics initiatives thus attempt to strengthen the athlete's resistance to doping even against what he may see as his own rational self-interest.

From a sociological standpoint, anti-doping work cannot exclusively or even primarily concentrate on measures that focus on the individual. Controls and penalties, as well as education by means of Fair Play initiatives, have a role to play, but they still remain inadequate if they are not accompanied by effective action on the structural level. *Because doping results from a social context, the context that produces doping must be changed*. Anti-doping work is, therefore, best seen as "context management" (Bette/Schimank 2000). This means that anti-doping measures must be coordinated with all of the social sectors that affect the risk profile of an athletic career. Collectively generated problems can only be solved in a collective manner. This applies to doping just as much as it applies to mad-cow disease or to ecological issues.

Here are some examples: Politicians should make use of their own resources by making funding dependent on anti-doping measures that are carried out at the federation level. This can involve decisions about payments and package deals. Corporate sponsors should direct their funding only to those federations that subject their athletes to unannounced testing. Meeting promoters should invite only those athletes who can show that they are in compliance with doping control regulations. The media should support this initiative by means of critical sports journalism. And the sporting public, despite the fact that it is not an organized collectivity, should support such initiatives by either attending or staying away from certain sporting events. These measures should be coordinated by a committee established for this purpose, since only in this way can organized sport learn how to give up the "convenient lawlessness" of doping and bring about changes in itself.

We are certainly aware of comparable crises which have managed to resolve themselves successfully. One need only think of the superpowers' "arms race" dating back to the 1950s, which by the 1980s had gradually been brought under control by means of arms control agreements. But even if such an example gives certain reasons for hope, we should not overlook the fact that the "arms race," for all of its perils, was actually less complex than the doping situation in two important ways. The "arms race" was the result of a bipolar relationship that was managed on both sides by the same military and political strategies. The doping situation, in contrast, comprises a wider range of actors and is affected by a greater number of strategies: sportive and political, those of corporations and the mass media, as well as by medical, legal, and educational perspectives. Nor should we overlook the spectators in the stadium who watch all of this happening. Another complicating factor is that certain subgroups, such as the media, are in fierce competition with each other and are not willing to engage in coordinated action.

It should be clear at the outset that every actor in this drama must be approached on his own terms. Only a respect for the complexity of the situation can make possible mutual understanding and successful collaboration. Limiting such efforts to the legal, economic, or sportive dimension is a short-cut that is also a prescription for failure. The different motives of the different actors must be made to converse with each other; in the last analysis, this discourse should aim at making it clear to the elite sport subculture that doping no longer pays.

Another thing that is needed is *an intelligent way to connect how the individual and how the sports community regulate their respective behaviors.* Organized sport must learn more than it has to date about how to be an appropriate milieu for the drug-free athlete. Politicians, corporations, the public, and the mass media should also realize how they too are a part of the doping problem. At this time, these parties do not seem to have much insight into their own involvement. Quite to the contrary: sponsors, political paymasters, the mass media, and the public defend themselves vigorously against the idea that they have anything to do with doping. They wash their innocent hands, claim that others are responsible for the problem, and thereby contribute to maintaining the doping system into the foreseeable future.

[Translated by John Hoberman]

References

Bette, Karl-Heinrich und Uwe Schimank, 1995: Doping im Hochleistungssport. Anpassung durch Abweichung. Frankfurt am Main: Suhrkamp Verlag.

Bette, Karl-Heinrich und Uwe Schimank, 1996: Coping mit Doping: die Sportverbände im Organisationsstreß. In: Sportwissenschaft 26. Jg., Heft 4, 357-382.

Bette, Karl-Heinrich und Uwe Schimank, 2000: Doping als Konstellationsprodukt. Eine soziologische Analyse. In: Michael Gamper, Jan Mühlethaler und Felix Reidhaar (Hrsg.), Doping. Spitzensport als gesellschaftliches Problem. Zürich: Verlag Neue Zürcher Zeitung, 91-112.

Hirsch, Fred, 1980: Social Limits to Growth. London: Routledge.

Perrow, Charles, 1984: Normal Accidents. New York: Basic Books.

CHAPTER 6

DOPING DILEMMAS AND PREVENTION STRATEGIES

Andreas Singler and Gerhard Treutlein

By now the problem of drug abuse in elite sport is well known. Discussions of the ethics of doping have become familiar exercises in ethical problem solving. These debates generally accomplish nothing, in that they have no effect on performance levels. Doping creates performance-related advantages for the athletes who use it even as it is officially frowned upon as a violation of elite sport's purported system of values. This situation confuses the public by creating a conflict between ethical values and the more pragmatic behavior represented by doping. This conflict pits obedience to the rules against sheer effectiveness. In the meantime, candid talk about doping has been essentially tabooed for many years as a violation of a certain code of conduct aimed at protecting the privacy of athletes. From this perspective, it is those who talk about drug use, not the dopers, who are to blame for the doping scandals that come to the attention of the public.

It would be wrong to assume that it is simply weakness of character that accounts for doping violations. The competitive sport system itself has a responsibility to promote ethical values for the purpose of educating the athletes. This is where sport pedagogy and sport sociology have something important to offer in the form of critical observations and analyses. But the ethical discussion must also be accompanied by policy initiatives undertaken by the responsible officials.

Competitive sport does not automatically produce positive qualities like independent thinking or maturity. The best insurance against doping is enabling athletes to think and behave independently and to reflect upon the consequences of their behaviour. Participants in competitive sport must be better prepared for this in the future, since they are likely to encounter the temptation of doping in the course of their careers as athletes, coaches, and doctors.

Ethical principles must be translated into action. The education of athletes can emphasize the importance of health and well-being. The coach-athlete relationship must be at the center of this endeavour. Coaches can play the essential role in preventing the emergence of a doping mentality.

This essay offers specific proposals for analysing doping dilemmas and proposes alternative courses of action. The most interesting aspect is the decline of performance levels from 1989 onwards (See Appendix 1). This is what happened in Germany, though it is true that on the international level China appears to have made up for the absence of the female athletes from the former East Germany (GDR). The standards produced by the female swimmers of the 1990s show that there is no decline in performance when no unannounced drug-tests are carried out during periods of training (see Appendix 2).

Developments in the endurance events indicate when the effects of EPO use began and that the case of Johan Mühlegg (Salt Lake, 2002) is not an isolated one (Singler & Treutlein 2000: 69-71). Despite performance declines we may assume that doping continues to play a significant role in elite sport.

The doping regulations and anti-doping laws of the 1960s, 1970s and 1980s had almost no impact on levels of performance. Neither political nor sports officials demonstrated the will to enact effective doping controls. Ethical discussions, hearings and commissions had no effect on performances. Other significant factors included the activities of some irresponsible sports physicians. Heinz Liesen, for example, told (West) German politicians in 1987 about having made world-class athletes out of mediocre athletes by means of "hormonal regulation" (Singler & Treutlein 2000: 303). We may assume that sports officials in the West were informed about doping and in some cases even encouraged it.

In West Germany, for example, most sports federations did not comply with the decision of the German Sports Association (DSB) to introduce drug-testing at competitions. The lack of adequate doping controls had the effect of allowing some doping to occur unchallenged by the sports system.

The determination to achieve improved performances at all costs existed in the West as well as in communist countries such as the GDR. Today many of the officials who were active during the recent doping decades continue to occupy leading positions in organised sport. This is particularly true at the international level, where it makes the campaign against doping very difficult. At the same time, some officials, such as the French anti-doping activist Claude-Louis Gallien, have come full circle to participate in anti-doping efforts.

Doping controls can be effective. It is an illusion, however, to think that increased controls will solve the doping problem. There is no one ideal way to eliminate doping, nor can doping be eradicated "once and for all." At the same time, fatalism or tolerance of doping are equally unacceptable.

The damage caused to elite sport due to doping-related drop-outs

The discussion concerning Germany's loss of sporting talent has entirely ignored doping as one possible reason for this problem. During the 1980's it became obvious that the high drop-out rate in West German elite sport was partly caused by doping (Singler & Treutlein 2001: 18-22). The need to take performance-enhancing drugs was one of the most important reasons that athletes considered retiring from elite sport. Those who did leave for this reason included not only athletes but also coaches, doctors, and sports administrators.

Doping-related retirements from elite sport happen for various reasons. An early example is the female shot-putters who were not nominated for the Olympic Games in 1972 in Munich although they had met the qualifying criteria. They had not, however, fulfilled the expectations of the (West German) Sports Association that was determined to use all available means, including anabolics. The result was that these athletes retired from shot-putting either immediately or after a short period of time; the coach, too, ended his career (Singler & Treutlein 2000: 76-80). This episode demonstrates how a sports federation can advise its athletes and coaches to use drugs without explicitly having to mention their performance-enhancing effects.

The damaging side-effects of highly effective drugs have contributed considerably to the drop-out problem. The most extreme example of a doping-related "drop-out" is the death of an athlete, as in the case of the heptathlete Birgit Dressel in 1987 (Singler & Treutlein 2000: 275-290).

Doping-related retirements have affected countries other than Germany. The number of athletes opposed to doping diminished due to a wave of retirements at all levels, whilst the influence of doping supporters increased proportionally and in absolute numbers. The world of sport lost many valuable people due to the self-destructive tendencies of an elite sport culture with its "winning-at-all-costs" mentality.

Doping creates medical dangers for women and girls

Equal legal and social status for men and women is one of the paramount aims of a modern, democratic society. The inherent logic of top-class sport, which is geared to short-term performance enhancement, can often prevent a responsible approach to the treatment of girls and women (Singler & Treutlein 2001: 89). Coaches who insist on keeping a tight rein on their athletes regard any attempt to reject a relationship of dependence, which is in fact neither justified nor necessary, as not "normal". When problems occur they attribute them solely to the athletes and not to themselves or the administrative arrangement. Female athletes who shun a relationship of dependence violate the coach's wish for control, predictability, dominance and power. A necessary prerequisite for change, should it be considered desirable, would be an analysis of the reasons that account for the theories and preferences of coaches. One might also ask why vacant positions are usually awarded to coaches who favour dependent relationships with their athletes.

Coaches should aim at slowly loosening the ties with their athletes and thus make themselves superfluous (Fulda 1992: 223). However, both the necessary training in this respect as well as control exercised by a professional association are lacking. The position of the coach within the present system makes it unlikely that educational ideals will be achieved (Treutlein 2001: 455). The activities of coaches – and particularly the activities of coaches who have specialised in training female athletes – take place in a social context that was not designed for educational purposes, but rather to achieve good performances. The "ethos of effectiveness" (Bette & Schimank 1995: 312) is still the predominant attitude in sport today. Coaches facing pressures to succeed are not equipped to deal with such issues as ethics, morality and educational requirements. A dependent, controllable and manipulable elite is the goal of many coaches and officials. It is a goal that is easier to achieve with women, as opposed to men, because of the gender stereotypes that still operate. Many coaches treat female athletes as if they were incapable of thinking and making decisions for themselves.

Adult male athletes generally take drugs on a voluntary basis, although there may be a degree of "encouragement" from those around them, as well. Female athletes, by contrast, who are generally more passive by nature, tend to be enticed into taking drugs. If priority is given to success and female athletes are treated as objects and if, as is the case, drug-taking by women is more effective than it is with men, it can come as no surprise that drug abuse assumes distinctive forms among top-class female athletes. Exaggerating a bit, one might say – taking into account stereotyped gender roles – that men take drugs, whereas women are given drugs (Singler & Treutlein 2001). Coaches play a much more prominent role in instigating and implementing the taking of drugs by female athletes than is the case with male athletes. Of course, the taking of performance-enhancing drugs by women in the GDR and the abuse that involved was even more brutal. The greater the dependence, the easier it is to manipulate women with the help of drugs.

The dilemma of value orientation versus pragmatic behaviour

Drug abuse has created advantages for those willing to achieve performances without regard for ethical standards. Drug abuse and the violation of rules constitute a strategy which inevitably leads into a dilemma (drug abuse = victory, while renunciation of drug abuse = defeat). A discrepancy exists between the commitment to self-imposed values on the one hand and pragmatic behaviour aimed at achieving success in sports on the other. Given the logic that prevails in elite sport today, values are not necessary for the achievement of success, so the preference is for a pragmatic approach. This leads to a disregard for the personality of the athlete and to the toleration of unfairness and deceit. The gulf between public proclamations about the pursuit of goals such as individual responsibility and self-determination and the preferred methods of success, which are dictated by the pressure to achieve, can only be bridged by resorting to such strategies as concealment and deliberately turning a blind eye. Unofficially, there is a tendency to eliminate from the system anyone who does not contribute to achieving top performances – as an athlete, coach, official or scientist, which is to say, anyone who does not clearly prefer a success-oriented approach.

Modern competitive sport thrusts individual athletes into dilemma situations that oppose the desire for clean, humane sports to expectations of success and improved performance. Such dilemma situations and devious behaviour are predictable. In the past, the system has made half-hearted attempts to restrain such developments. Concealment and the condoning of unethical behaviour were essential strategies for coping with this dilemma. Concealment indicates that there are taboos which exclude certain topics from public discussion (Hahn 1991: 88). For decades it has been common to talk about drug abuse in abstract terms and demand the prohibition of drugs, whereas talking about the realities of drug abuse has been taboo. The violation of the taboo was taken as a violation of a certain code of conduct and exerted pressure on those involved in the problem, since the prevailing code of silence was thereby threatened. According to the "pragmatic" view, it was not those taking drugs, but those talking about drugs, who were to blame for the embarrassment caused by doping scandals.

Experience teaches us that simply talking about ethics and social and educational objectives generally achieves nothing. The noble aims that are supposedly pursued in elite sport have been formulated in countless speeches and declarations, such as the one given at the 1996 Cologne Workshop that was sponsored by the Federal Institute of Sports Science and the German Sports Association Federal Committee for Basic and Advanced Training: "The work of coaches is subject to the general criteria that apply to any kind of educational responsibility for, and supervision of, athletes. The concept on which it must be based, therefore, is that of respect for individual human beings, their dignity and integrity." In other words, coaches should be specialists in handling people in a humane way.

It would be wrong to assume that it is simply weakness of character that accounts for why individuals violate their proclaimed values and goals. Given the way elite sport is structured at present, a "pragmatic" approach deviating from the ethical norm is only to be expected. The setting of standards may be proclaimed in fine speeches, but ultimately there is no practical follow-up. The dominance of expediency, i.e. success at any price, is reflected in the suppression of values and the preservation of double standards.

Competitive elite sport has a special responsibility towards athletes, and this includes the training and selection of coaches. Observing and reflecting on their own activities and those of others is essential to enable coaches to handle any dilemmas that might arise and to ensure that values and the pursuit of educational objectives in top-class sport are given the status they deserve. Expediency and pragmatism are all too compatible with the logic of the system, while ethical values exercise a restraining influence.

Sport pedagogy, which means providing codes of conduct and values; and sport sociology, which means observation and reflection above all of blind spots, can make a useful contribution here in the form of critical observation and reflection on decisions, activities and processes. They can point to blind spots in the way that competitive sport sees itself, which is particularly important in the case of the relationship between male coaches and female athletes.

This ethics discussion is necessary but useless unless it is accompanied by efforts on the administrative level that can affect the athletic environment and the education of athletes. The first task of effective prevention is to show how doping practices arise and how divergent behaviour is learned as well as which excuses are used to justify these behaviours. Effective counter-arguments must be formulated. The tyranny of sheer performance must be resisted as much as possible. This can only be achieved when the athlete is treated as a subject and not as a consumer product. The education and selection of coaches must be a primary objective. Coaches usually have the greatest influence on the decisions athletes make about doping. If coaches stand firm against doping, the probability that a doping mentality will arise is low. If the coach is not convincing, then one should not be surprised when athletes dope themselves.

In sports federations and clubs today there are many officials, coaches, and doctors who were there during the "great" era of doping and who participated in the doping culture. With the exception of France, there is no evidence, either on the national or international level, of real determination to do something about doping in a thorough and consistent way. Moreover, the sort of ani-doping work that targets only the athlete and restricts itself to a "negative pedagogy" of doping controls and penalties will always be an inadequate strategy.

Since doping cannot be eliminated, dilemma situations inevitably arise. It therefore seems urgently necessary that these be identified at all levels and that strategies to deal with them be worked out. The following levels have to be taken into account:

Figure 1: Multi-level model of complex doping prevention.

Level		Measures	Theoretical foundations
5th	International (UN, EU, IOC, IAAF etc.)	WADA/rules: reduction of structural pressures, e.g., raising of the minimum age, reducing the number of major competitions, controls, penalties	sociology of sport, political science, systems theory
4th	State/society	Medicine, law, developmental regulations (e.g. norms, discussions, professional support), anti-doping agency	sociology of sport, political science, systems theory
3rd	Sports associations	Sports regulations, setting standards, selection rules (e.g., choosing coaches)	sociology of sport, political science, systems theory, psychology of sport
2nd	Association/ athletic environment	Rigorousness of selection (e.g. coaches according to their pedagogical suitability), doping-resistant environment, improvement in counseling services	Sport pedagogy, sport didactics, psychology of learning, criminal sociology
1st	Athlete	Development of the individual's ability to resist (arguments, sense of responsibility, decision skills), preparation for dilemma situations, information available for young athletes	Sport pedagogy, sport didactics, psychology of learning

It is important to distinguish between structural and educational preventive measures. Structural measures are the responsibility of international and national sport organisations and pertain to the athletic environment as well as the schools. At the same time, we must recognize that responsibility for the doping problem is not just the fault of the system but also includes individual deviance and weakness of character on the part of individual athletes. It is the very complexity of doping that makes reliance on doping controls and penalties an inadequate strategy.

General suggestions

1. Leadership positions in international sports organisations must be occupied by people of integrity who are unencumbered by associations with the doping culture; for example, Manuela di Centa, an athlete representative on the IOC, should be excluded on the grounds that she has been implicated in doping.
2. Dopers have a great advantage over those who oppose doping, according to the scientists and academics who study the doping phenomenon. Langauge barriers confine much knowledge about doping to the national communities in which it occurs. For this reason, the translation of the relevant literature into other languages is of crucial importance.
3. International conferences should bring together sports sociologists, sport pedagogues, and sport psychologists to explore the difficulties involved in combating doping.
4. Permanent committees should clarify the responsibility for and co-ordination of doping prevention measures at the national and international levels.
5. There should be a catalogue of anti-doping strategies for both organised sports and non-organised sports.

The available literature for the "positive training" of athletes should be catalogued. Proposals by Singler & Treutlein, Bette & Schimank, as well as the current French, Swiss, and Italian materials would be useful and would require translation. This would prevent much redundant effort.

Suggestions regarding educational measures

Here we must distinguish between a "negative pedagogy" and a "positive pedagogy":

Doping prevention

	"Negative training" (negative pedagogy – suppression)	"Positive training" (positive pedagogy – prevention)
Aims	Suppression of the phenomenon	Ability of the subjects to resist the temptation to dope
Measures	Controls, penalties	Sense of responsibility and an ability to make decisions

What we are calling "negative pedagogy" is already well developed in the form of laws, controls and penalties, while "positive pedagogy" has been neglected. The IOC and the international federations appear to feel that they have no responsibility in this area, and the same applies to Germany.

Attitudes toward the doping problem at the higher levels of elite sport can appear quite cynical. Similarly, the attitudes of sponsors such as states, corporations, and military establishments can be equally cynical when there is an exclusive fixation on sporting success. The idea that elite sport can by itself enable athletes to think independently about doping is quite implausible. If anything, elite sport participation tends to encourage athletes' dependence on authority figures within the sports milieu. The best insurance against doping is to enable athletes to think and behave independently and to reflect upon the short- and long-term consequences of their behaviour. Anti-doping education can also include training children and adolescents to think for themselves about doping issues.

The observation that social learning takes place primarily in small groups suggests that coaches can have a greater influence than the parents of competitive athletes due to the strong relationship that exists between coach and athlete. Coaches can thus play the essential role in preventing the development of a doping mentality. Treutlein, Janalik & Hanke (19964) argue that young athletes should, for example, be able to weigh the pros and cons of proposals to legalise doping or to employ steroids for the purpose of "regeneration."

Treutlein et al (19964) give the following example of a predicament in which young athletes can find themselves.

You are a junior racing cyclist in training. You are constantly being confronted by fellow athletes who tell you that without doping you will not have a chance to make it to the top of your sport. You hear similar remarks during conversations at competitions. You get specific advice about which drugs you should take and which doctors will take care of you.
A) You don't listen and carry on as before, while other cyclists who once finished behind you now finish ahead of you at competitions.
B) You write down the name of the drug and the address of the doctor.
C) You register a protest with the federation officials.

You inform a journalist you know about the suggestions you have been getting from your fellow athletes. (Singler & Treutlein 2001: 256).

Conclusion

In 1993 the prominent German scientist and anti-doping activist Werner Franke warned about the dangers of gene doping at a meeting of the German Athletics Federation (DLV) in Erfurt and called for preventive measures. At this time, however, preventive measures against the threat of genetic engineering do not exist. Elite sport remains essentially defenseless against such grave threats to its fundamental integrity.

References

Berendonk, B.: Doping. Von der Forschung zum Betrug. Rororo, Hamburg 1992.

Bette, K.H. & Schimank, U.: Doping im Hochleistungssport. Edition Suhrkamp, Frankfurt 1995.

Bette, K.H. et al.: Biographische Dynamiken im Leistungssport. Möglichkeiten der Dopingprävention im Jugendalter. Strauß, Köln 2002.

Fulda, B. (1992): Mädchen im Spitzensport – Pädagogische Überlegungen und geschlechtsspezifische Perspektiven. In: Brennpunkt der Sportwissenschaft 6, 2, p. 218-229.

Hahn, A. (1991): Rede- und schweigeverbote. In: Kölner Zeitschrift für Soziologie und Sozialpsychologie, 43, 86-105.

Houlihan, B.: Dying to win. Doping in sport and the development of anti-doping policy. European Council, Strasbourg 1999.

Laure, P. (Ed.): Dopage et société. Ellipse, Paris 2000.

Spitzer, G.: Doping in der DDR. Ein historischer Überblick zu einer konspirativen Praxis. Strauss, Köln 1998.

Singler, A. & Treutlein, G.: Doping im Spitzensport. Sportwissensschaftliche Analysen zur nationalen und internationalen Leistungsentwicklung. Meyer&Meyer, Aachen 2000.

Singler, A. & Treutlein, G.: Doping – von der Analyse zur Prävention. Meyer&Meyer, Aachen 2001.

Treutlein, G. (1985): Zum Problem von Abhängigkeit und Fremdbestimmung in der Frauenleichtathletik. In: N. Müller, D.Augustin & B.Hunger (Eds.): Frauenleichtathletik. Kongressbericht. Niedernhausen, 404 – 409.

Treutlein, G. (1994): Zwischen Wertorientierung und Zweckrationalität. Handlungsdilemmata im Leistungssport. In: K.H. Bette (Ed.): Doping im Leistungssport – sozialwissenschaftlich betrachtet. Stuttgart, 153 – 166.

Treutlein, G. (2001): Trainerrolle und Professionalisierung. In: H. Haag & A. Hummel (Eds.): Handbuch Sportpädagogik. Schorndorf 2001, 455 – 460.

Treutlein, G., Janalik, H. & Hanke, U. (1989): Wie Trainer wahrnehmen, fühlen, denken und handeln. Köln.

Treutlein, G., Janalik, H. & Hanke, U. (1996[4]): Wie Sportlehrer wahrnehmen, fühlen, denken und handeln. Köln.

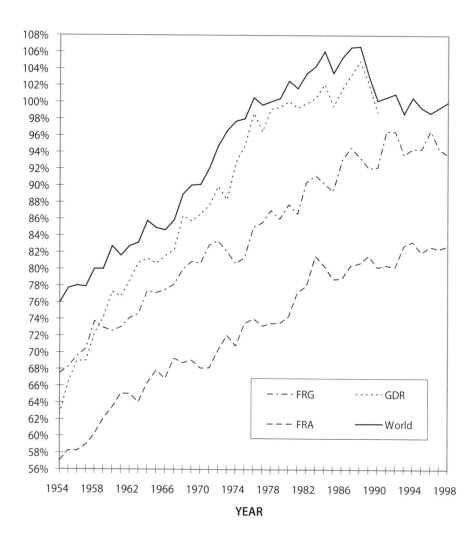

APPENDIX 1:

The development of the shot putting results between 1954 and 1998 based on the average distances of the top three female competitors; the results of 1998 are taken as 100% (cf. Singler & Treutlein, 2000, 149).

ANDREAS SINGLER & GERHARD TREUTLEIN

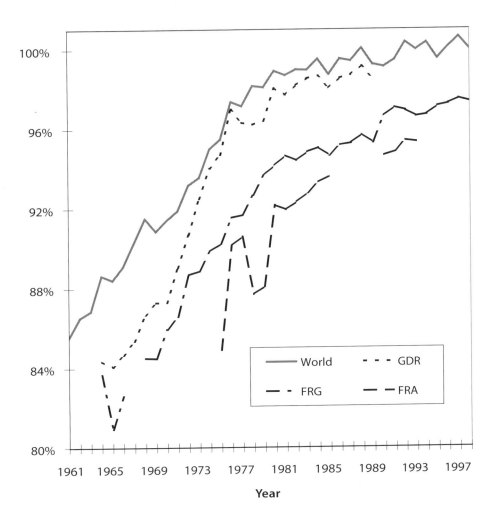

APPENDIX 2:

The delevepment of the swimming results between 1961 andf 1998 based on the average distances of the top three female competitors; the results of 1998 are taken as 100% (cf. Singler & Treutlein, 2000, 70).

CHAPTER 7

THE PREVENTION OF DOPING IN SPORT: PROTECTING ADOLESCENT ATHLETES

Patrick Laure

The prevention of doping is by now a familiar subject that has been publicly debated since the 1950s. The effectiveness of this campaign, however, remains very questionable.

I would like to propose that we revisit this topic keeping in mind the questions that are being posed by the "International Network for Humanistic Doping Research":

(1) What are the objectives of doping prevention programmes? Are they
   (a)   to reduce the number of athletes who practice doping?
   (b)   to reduce the number of those who begin to practice doping?
   (c)   to limit the number of those who are moving toward systematic doping after having experimented with doping products?
   (d)   to reduce the health risks associated with doping products?
   (e)   to rehabilitate former users of doping products?

(2) Which methods should be used to achieve these objectives, especially when dealing with adolescents?

(3) How can we be sure that these objectives have been achieved, and if they have not been, why did they fail?

Prevention

Preventive measures anticipate behaviours that a specific social group has judged to be problematic because they violate fundamental values. The objective is to prevent these behaviours from occurring, or at least to limit their negative effects.

Fundamental values

For a social group such fundamental values may be freedom, security, equality, and health, to name just a few. Prevention presupposes values that are worth defending and that derive from a code of ethics. Prevention is thus focused on respect for the individual. Preventive actions that are not based on ethical standards amount to no more than manipulation.

Behaviour

Prevention affects behaviour and can change it over time. This means that we must understand the factors that determine behaviour and the environment in which it takes place. We must also understand that we are dealing with "the individual" and thus with ideas about human dignity and respect for the human person. Here ethics occupies a primary role.

Judging problem behaviour

Prevention programmes are irrelevant unless the behaviour in question is regarded as presenting a problem. If this is not the case, then society will see no reason to take preventive measures against it. Doping presents us with a situation of this kind. Numerous opinion polls, even if we concede the limitations of this kind of data, suggest that the general public believes that doping only concerns professional athletes such as cyclists and footballers. At the same time, the low percentage of positive drug tests, which average between one and three percent annually, reassures the sports community that doping affects only a very small fraction of athletes, and that it need not be a matter of major concern.

When prevention does appear to fail, the problem behaviour is sanctioned in a way that is assumed to be proportionate to the damage that has been done to the fundamental values of society. It is ethics that justifies the punishment. In the case of doping, sanctions are directed against the consumers of drugs. Those who are sanctioned may be consumers of so-called recreational drugs; they may be athletes who use doping products that appear on official lists of banned substances; or they may be traffickers who sell these illegal products. Prevention and the imposing of sanctions are the two necessary and complementary ways to regulate doping.

From doping to doping behaviour

By definition, athletic doping involves a very small fraction of the general population (those who practice sports) and only a small fraction of the pharmaceutical products that are obtainable on various markets, namely, the »banned« substances. These illicit substances appear on a list formulated by the Medical Commission of the International Olympic Committee (IOC).

Doping thus defined may be considered a violation of the rules of sport and, in countries such as France and Belgium, as violations of national anti-doping laws. The problem is that this definition, while useful for formulating sanctions (because it distinguishes between what is allowed and what is forbidden), is not appropriate for the purpose of prevention.

To illustrate this point let us imagine the following situation: You are young athletes and I am your coach. We have just been talking about doping and because doping threatens your health and is contrary to the ideal of »fair play« – the twin pillars of the anti-doping campaign – I have just convinced you that you should not consume any of the products that are on the banned list. But someone else – another coach, a parent, perhaps a team- mate – could tell you something quite different: »So, you've understood … You must not use these products. On the other hand, you *can* use all of the products that are not on the list: iron, megadoses of vitamins, creatine, tranquillisers, anti-depressants, etc. Since they are not on the list, using them does not count as doping."

And this person would be right, despite the fact that using these substances can often be dangerous to your health and might even contradict certain ethical standards.

A second example: You are still adolescents, but this time you are studying for an examination at school. Well, why not use all of the products on the banned list? After all, you are not athletes. Suffice it to say that adolescents do not think this situation makes much sense.

Doping-behaviour (1)

It is for this reason that in 1997 I proposed the concept of "doping-behaviour." This concept has since been adopted by a number of publications and has found a role in prevention work in France at the national level. The concept of doping-behaviour was proposed to add some nuance to a concept of doping that is too simplistic to be useful in the field of prevention. A second objective was to help define "drug-taking," which many authors, and particularly Anglo-Saxon commentators, *do not* distinguish from "doping." "Drug-taking" is another form of substance abuse, but unlike "doping," the objective is rather sensation-seeking, whether this is for recreational purposes, or to forget one's problems, or to break the law, or to engage in risk-taking.

Doping-behaviour is by definition the use of a substance for the purpose of improving one's ability to confront an obstacle, real or imagined, and which is perceived as real by the drug-taker or by the people around him. In the case of this definition the nature of the substance is of little importance. The "obstacle" can take different forms: a sports competition, a school examination, a job interview, etc. The obstacle may be real, such as a very difficult examination, or an obstacle that is essentially imagined, such as taking a driving test or giving a speech in public. In addition, this imaginary obstacle is perceived as real not only by the drug-taker but also by the people around him, such as parents, team-mates, colleagues on the job, etc. Finally, "performance" as it is construed here is not necessarily associated with a sporting event. The concept of performance is inherent in the person's customary physical and social environment. For example, high performance for certain mothers would mean being able to "manage" the youngest child's fifteen friends during his or her birthday party.

Doping thus seems to be a particular kind of doping behaviour in so far as it concerns a limited population (those who engage in sports) along with a limited number of products (the list of doping substances) and the regulation of these products (which forbid it).

Doping-behaviour (2)

The fundamental point of the concept of doping-behaviour is precisely that it focuses on behaviours that we want to better understand.

A consumption-behaviour

Doping-behaviour is a form of substance use. Here "consumption" can be subdivided into use, abuse, and dependence: three terms that are frequently used when talking about addictions. Thus, a link can be established between the concepts of "doping-behaviour" and "consumption."

A determined behaviour

The determining factors of this consumption-behaviour that aims at improving performance can be grouped into three categories:

(a) *Predisposing factors* (the indirect causes of the behaviour): these factors are specific to the individual (sex, age, socio-professional category) and/or are external (the influence of parental role-models, etc.).

(b) *Driving factors* (the direct causes of the behaviour), such as conflict, previous failure, etc., aggravated by risk factors (fear of rejection, previous use of a substance, suggestibility, peer-pressure, etc., and counter-balanced by protective factors such as self-esteem, independence, etc.

(c) *Triggering factors* which come into play when a person who is predisposed and has been "driven" by certain factors encounters a substance while the protective factors are unable to outweigh or overcome his risk factors. This contact can occur when a substance is offered, or when a third person proposes the use of a product, or in response to a request, where it is the individual himself who "drives" his own consuming behaviour (directly if he procures the drug for himself, indirectly if he asks someone else to get it for him).

Risk-taking behaviour

Risk-taking behaviour can be defined as a type of experimental behaviour that may lead to undesirable effects on the health of the individual or of the people around him. This behaviour is located on the boundary of »the permitted« and »the forbidden.« It also marks the boundary that separates »the known« (present state of the individual) from the »unknown« (consequences of his actions for who he is).

By engaging in this kind of behaviour the individual weighs and discards the significance of the social limits (by breaking the rules) and deals with his own limits (by manifesting his capacity to surpass himself). One should learn to recognise the potential danger involved in this kind of behaviour. However, knowledge of the risk involved does not always lead to the individual's giving up the dangerous behaviour. For example, in a study carried out on 138 male body-builders, 87% of the anabolic steroid users thought that the products were dangerous, but only 11% reported they would stop taking them on account of their undesirable side-effects.

In the case of adolescent athletes, some research suggests that they may be more inclined than non-athletes to engage in risk-taking behaviour. This is even more likely when they are deeply involved in their sport. It has recently been observed, for example, that adolescents who are engaged in sport for more than eight hours a week experience a higher rate of automobile accidents, theft (either from shops or from relatives), fighting incidents (including group violence, bullying and violence directed against individuals), other violent incidents (physical assault, the use of weapons, vandalism of public and private property) and consumption of illegal substances (synthetic drugs, heroin, cocaine) than is the case among other adolescents. In addition, adolescents who use substances such as anabolic steroids in order to improve their performances seem to engage in risk-taking behaviour more often than non-consumers. In some cases, then, there seems to be a link between risk-taking behaviour and doping-behaviour. The precise nature of this link remains unclear.

Behaviour for the purpose of preventing failure

If an individual takes products to enhance performance, it is because he wants to have every advantage when confronting the challenge. The individual wants to give himself every possible opportunity *not* to fail whatever the situation involves, be it an examination, a job interview, or a sports competition. In other words, he is trying to avoid personal failure, a term that carries ominous implications in societies that produce both exclusion and failure on a large scale. Doping-behaviour is, therefore, behaviour that is intended to prevent failure.

The prevention of doping-behaviour therefore raises questions about the legitimacy of interventions that are designed to stop people from engaging in behaviours which allow them to overcome obstacles and thus avoid failure or at least limit its effects. This is all the more significant in a society that exposes increasing numbers of people to the risk of experiencing personal failure.

The prevention of doping-behaviour

Why engage in preventive measures? Before we can envisage the methods to be used, we need to determine why we should implement prevention programmes in the first place. In the wider society, for example, virtually no one worries about the use of drugs to improve performance. For this reason, doping-behaviour should be seen as:

- a grass roots demand coming from rank-and-file athletes including adolescents;
- behaviour that is seen as necessary and that has been identified by experts after performing diagnostic studies;
- a response that has been legitimated by decision-makers for a variety of reasons – economics, politics, security considerations – but which is not necessarily based on a demand or a real need;
- a combination of two or even all three of the factors mentioned above.

Any of these options is in itself legitimate and can thus justify a potential intervention assuming it is realistic.

Doping-prevention up to this point

Since 1960 initiatives aimed at doping-prevention have been undertaken at the request of international authorities such as the Council of Europe and UNESCO. These programs, aimed primarily at dissuading young competitors from using drugs, proved to be largely ineffective. One likely reason for this failure is that these programs have relied on tactics that offer little prospect for success by virtue of the fact that they either do not target appropriate mediating mechanisms or do not have a sufficient impact on mediating mechanisms that are correctly targeted. Examples of such failed tactics include: using scare tactics, claiming that drugs do not enhance performance, emphasising the role of ethics in sport, and increasing young athletes' knowledge of drugs.

It is now widely recognised that prevention programs produce their effects by altering protective and risk factors that account for drug use. Some recent studies have shown that health education aimed at young athletes can have a meaningful effect on doping prevention.

Prevention aimed at adolescents

All forms of intervention that aim to prevent doping-behaviour must take the individual into consideration. Prevention is an evolving process that must constantly be adapted to the individual and to his or her social group and cultural origins, to changing moral values and thus to the degree of concern that results from problematic behaviours. At the same time, it would be simplistic to focus entirely on the individual. Prevention must also target and change the social environment, as well. Finally, the essential point for any prevention program is *not to forget to involve* the adolescents themselves who must participate in the decision-making process. This approach is predicated on the young person's freely accepting the value system that prevention represents.

Conclusion

Health education and the promotion of self-esteem have proven to be the most effective approach to the prevention of doping-behaviour. This success derives from the fact that this approach allows adolescents to take responsibility for the decisions they make about how they are going to behave. The next problem concerns the feasibility of applying this approach to the real world of adolescent sports. It must be applied over a long period of time and involve many participants in the overall process. That is why the prevention of doping-behaviour should be integrated into the general education of adolescents.

CHAPTER 8

A LENINIST MONSTER:
COMPULSORY DOPING AND PUBLIC POLICY IN THE G.D.R. AND THE LESSONS FOR TODAY

Giselher W. Spitzer

The compulsory doping system of the former German Democratic Republic was an inhuman project that invites polemical analysis of its medical crimes against the young athletes who fell under its influence. This essay aims, however, at providing a historical and sociological reconstruction of GDR doping for the purpose of examining what it can teach us about doping in elite sport today. State-sponsored doping in the GDR is presented here as a massive violation of human rights that took place in the heart of Europe. The frequently invoked comparison with the medical crimes of the Nazis is imprecise but not without a certain relevance to the field of medical ethics. The purpose of the essay can be described as follows:

- First, I offer an explanation of how doping on this scale could happen and then proceed to examine compulsory doping as a systematic public policy;
- Second, I suggest what free and pluralistic societies can learn about doping as a social system, even if the GDR dictatorship no longer exists today.

Elite sport in the GDR was invented and controlled by the communist Socialist Unity Party (SED). After 1945 the Communist party (KPD, later SED) appeared to be governing sports organisations in a democratic way; internally, however, the strategy was to maintain control of everything in sports at every level. The traditional (democratically organised) sports clubs were abolished. The GDR developed in their place its own system of public sports organizations:

- A minority of these functionaries came from the Communist movement but had never before been connected with sports. Sport development at this time expedited careers by producing good results, not by promoting values in sport.
- The members of the generation that built sport in the GDR were in most cases former "Hitlerjungen" (Hitler Youth, or HJ).

One high-ranking Nazi who went into the sports field had been the personal assistant of a provincial governor (Gau-Führer) and leader of a "Hitlerjugend-Streife," a Nazi gang that was vested with the full rights of regular policemen.

This individual – let us call him "Manfred" – persecuted young members of the workers movement who refused to salute the Nazi flag. These brave boys were beaten by "Manfred" and his political gang and in some cases severely injured. As police reports show, this even happened after the Nazi surrender in May 1945.

"Manfred", a member of the NSDAP, sought out young members of the SS and the Waffen-SS. He did not fight against the Russians, but rather fled when it became clear that the Nazis' days were numbered. He then began to build the sports organisation of the formally independent but communist-controlled "Freie Deutsche Jugend" ("FDJ"). One FDJ leader of that era was Erich Honecker, the last unelected leader of the SED. "Manfred" started a career, bringing his HJ-friends with him. That led to anger and opposition from other members of the SED who had been beaten by the very same "Manfred" before 1945. In 1952 he was made secretary of state for physical culture and sport for the GDR.

This man's real name was Manfred Ewald, later an elected member of the Central Committee of the SED and, of course, head of the GDR sports organization and of its NOC.[1]

From 1961 to 1988 Ewald was personally responsible for doping in the GDR. We will interpret his brand of doping as a Leninist strategy that was pursued without any consideration for ethical or health concerns. From 1948 on the political aim was to defeat the Western sporting nations, the first priority being the Federal Republic of Germany (FRG).

The elite sport system of the GDR

We will next describe the hidden professional system of GDR sport from the critical perspective of social science. The elite sport system integrated doping into its operations. Performance-enhancing drugs were not optional additions to training, coaching and science, but were rather a required part of all planning from early on.

How can we account for the numerous violations of human rights that were committed by highly qualified, academically educated coaches, medical doctors and academic researchers? We will find some of the answers by applying professional ethics to this problem.[2] That could be useful, given that athletes' abuse of pharmaceutical products continues to be a problem in elite sport.

The historical background of East German high-performance sport should be seen in relation to the relatively smooth functioning of the sports establishment in the Federal Republic of Germany (let us call it "the West"). In this context I would like to make two points:

(1) Characteristic of Eastern European societies in the post-war era is the remarkably slow passing of *social time*. This is particularly apparent in the East German system of sport, with its special sociological and socio-historical features. To the external observer, this system appeared to follow the process of modernization, but in reality it continued to represent an obsolete, regressive and inhuman social arrangement.

Even though East German high-performance sport attained a higher degree of differentiated self-organization than any other Western European sport system, it was only able to create the illusion of keeping up with the growing demands made upon it. This in itself is both remarkable and an example of an illusory "progressive" policy. It contrasts with the more credible progressive policies of the FRG since the 1960s. Staying in touch with the changing attitudes of the athletes, ensuring greater inclusion through the popularization of integrated social sport programs, and maintaining an openness towards new types of sport are typical examples of this more enlightened approach.

(2) In the general overview, I will refer to the structural elements of East German Olympic sport, which was and always had been professionally organized.

The elite sport system of the GDR was a secret operation. Important directives from the sports leadership were sent by encrypted telegrams to the offices of the sports clubs and regional organizations, which operated under cover of secrecy. Many of their practices, in fact, would have incurred jail sentences under East German law.

A second aspect of GDR doping involved a special kind of a social contract. We may call this a politically controlled professional sport culture that offered life-long employment as one of its benefits.

The procedure for selecting the most promising athletic material went as follows. The first stage was an (ethically dubious) analysis of the entire German youth population: approximately 60,000 children were selected according to scientific criteria and their interest in particular types of sport was encouraged by a coach. They did not make their own decisions; since the candidate had no freedom in the choice of his or her sport. Only about 40% found their way into their chosen sports in the traditional manner, through personal interest or private consultation with athletes or coaches. Training took place in one of about 1,800 special centers.

Through rigorous selection, the most promising 10,000 athletes were accepted yearly into the 2nd level, these athletes were assigned to "sport clubs" and educated in "child and youth sport schools."

Those who did not "keep up" fell "into a hole". Why? Because the GDR decided to save money rather than provide this large group with organized competitive leagues as had always been the case in the days of the Weimar Republic. The majority of those selected reported having had negative experiences with organized sport.

Those who belonged to the so-called "second circle" or to the national teams (the "first circle") or to the 3rd level (high-performance training in the sports club) could rise into the ranks of the top 2000 athletes.

In the final analysis, then, only the most resilient 3% of the athletes pre-selected from the overall analysis of the entire East German youth cohort were selected. No other sector of East German society offered a comparable system of promotion.

As for the material resources of the GDR sport system, the following has become clear. Despite the guarantees made in the constitution and by the Communist ruling party, the lion's share of the financial resources did not go to large-scale sport programs to benefit the general population, but rather to high-performance sport. This is one reason, among others, for the lower participation rates in sport, that still persist in the states of the former East Germany, which are fully two-thirds lower than those in the West.

The exact figures are difficult to obtain. At the time, they were kept strictly confidential, and they can only be reconstructed by consulting the "even more confidential" files kept by the Ministry of State Security.

Assuming that, in high-performance sport alone, at least 4,700 professional coaches were employed, we can calculate that at least 500,000,000 D-Marks were paid to them in salary. The 1,000 medical doctors in professional sport would have cost 200,000,000 D-marks, and the 5,000 administrators *and* functionaries another 400,000,000 D-marks. The costs for research and doping are unknown.

As of 1952 professional status in sport could be achieved while bypassing amateur status. Relief from work obligations was achieved by paying above-average wages premiums included. This was arranged through the factories or through the state via the sport organizations. If the athlete conformed to the political rules of conduct, additional sums would be paid after the end of his or her career. This effectively guaranteed a high degree of political correctness among the athletes. (The author knows of many such cases.[3]) In addition, from the 1960s onward, there was guaranteed education and, of particular importance today, life-long employment. By signing on as a professional athlete, one initiated this sort of career. This agreement amounted to a "muzzle contract" which had nothing whatsoever to do with contractual freedom and self-determination.

- GDR athletes were exceptionally well-paid civil servants with a guaranteed career and the obligation to withhold information about the daily practices of athletic life. They were also forbidden to have contact with any persons or organizations not affiliated with the government.

A characteristic feature of the daily life of the athlete was the rigorous control of every aspect by the Socialist Unity Party and the Secret Service, which effectively stifled all capacity for reform. Informally known as the 'Stasi', the terrorist Secret Service of the GDR used approximately 3,000 volunteer agents ("inoffizielle Mitarbeiter", called IM's in German, or "unofficial collaborators") to maintain control of the elite sport community. Perfecting a system of absolute control in internal affairs was as much the goal of the Ministry for State Security as was the espionage directed at West Germany and at the "traitors to the Republic" who had emigrated to the West.

The Stasi's operations in the West reached as far as the West German sports ministry and the presidium of its National Olympic Committee. The contents of confidential discussions regularly found their way from these organizations to East Berlin, often as soon as the night after the meeting had occurred. On the other hand, no records of Western espionage within the GDR sports establishment have come to light.

The functionaries and committees of the Socialist Unity Party (SED) exerted their influence on all sectors of society. The sport system, for example, was actually directed by a secret and unofficial party commission within the Central Committee of the SED, called the "competitive sports commission of the GDR," which bypassed the official channels.

Secret and medically hazardous training methods were covered up and only discussed with athletes in exceptional situations. The resulting medical harm was covered up as effectively as possible, which increased the likelihood of permanent damage. Spot checks show that these medical consequences were considerably more serious than has been reported. For example, the "magic" limit of 20% for the purpose of calculating the degree of disability for insurance purposes was only rarely exceeded, since one percent more would have invoked the category called "serious disability resulting from sport" in the official records. This lead to lying about insurance to the disadvantage of the athletes, and this too was organised by the terrorist Secret Service. Doping agents and methods were euphemistically referred to as "supportive medications." The historical development of the doping program can be described as follows:

- The *Pre-Anabolic phase* – that involved the various 'classic' stimulants dating from the 1950s;
- The *Anabolic phase* – involving the massive abuse of anabolic steroids (around 10 kg or 2 million tablets a year) dating from 1966;
- The *Blood Doping* phase dating from 1972;
- The *Post-Anabolic phase* beginning with the ethically deplorable administration of cerebral and peptide hormones from the period between 1973 and 1980;
- The abuse of natural and synthetic hormones since 1983. The first medically documented use of human growth hormone on an athlete in the GDR took place without the knowledge of the test subject, a professional cyclist.

Human experimentation was a common aspect of the "central planning" of the criminal medicine that was practised in East German elite sport. This group of at least 1500 persons was involved in "research" and "applications," overlapping at times with certain special interests of the terrorist Secret Service. All of this took place under the supervision of the state-run "Sports Medicine Service of the GDR" (SMD), with the express knowledge of high functionaries such as Erich Honecker or Minister of Sport Prof. Guenter Erbach. The administration included a man whose past was perhaps more heavily compromised by Nazi involvement than anyone else in the GDR government, namely, Manfred Ewald. He became the first Minister of Sport in 1952 and was later named President of the DTSB (German Gymnastics and Sports Association). Ewald was responsible for "special measures" ("Sondermassnahmen") such as injecting male hormones into women, while "specially commissioned agents" supervised the preparations for Olympic Games.

From 1972 onward 2,000 male and female athletes were doped annually in conformity with the central plan, the overwhelming majority without their knowledge or their legal consent. By my estimate, the victims subjected to these assaults on their health number around 10,000. The destructive physical effects of doping can be determined through research and confirmed in court proceedings. Among the approximately 500 officially doped GDR athletes, effects such as cardiac muscle damage and liver damage are to be expected, or what I have called *damage to the phenotype*. Effects on the germ line resulting in fetal handicaps may have been higher than in the population as a whole, independent of the degree of steroid abuse. I have called this effect *damage to the genotype*. Today we see a greater than average number of crippled or handicapped children in the children of athletes once active in cycling, swimming and the strength disciplines, in particular. In one year, for example, cyclists belonging to one club had three severely handicapped babies.

Approximately 25% of the anabolic steroids were experimental substances that will not be checked for side-effects until the affected athletes apply for retirement benefits. Their effects remain unknown, as these substances have never been tested. According to official GDR research, exactly one-third of the women and girls suffered serious gynecological damage. My interviews with many female former athletes show that, on the contrary, such damage was suffered in almost every single case.

We must take the problems of the thousands of drugged athletes who once competed for the GDR seriously. Take, for example, some of the cases tried in German courts in recent years. Of the nine witnesses tested for physical disabilities related to doping who testified in the "Dynamo" trial, one had already been suffering from liver cancer, which would have remained undiagnosed but for the medical examination ordered by the court. If the tumour grows and blocks a blood vessel, the life of this victim is in danger. She is herself a medical doctor who never considered this possibility, because she was not aware of the risk.

"Double doping"

It is interesting to note that before the 1988 Seoul Games the GDR leadership had secret plans for achieving the No. 1 ranking among the world's sporting nations. And why not? After all East German cheating methods had been quite successful at the 1980 Moscow Games. Here dozens of Olympic medals were the result of "perfect" doping methods that involved what the East Germans called "double doping."

"Double" doping means that, in addition to the "normal" abuse of anabolic steroids during the training period, one achieves a maximum dosage while avoiding a positive test. The GDR was highly skilled in applying this form of cheating which yielded the following results:

In track & field: 9 gold, 2 silver and 3 bronze medals (8 athletes); in skiing: 1 Olympic gold medal (team); in cycling: 1 silver medal; in judo: 3 bronze medals won by three athletes; in swimming: 10 gold, 7 silver- and 2 bronze medals won by 7 athletes.

In summary, no fewer than 20 GDR gold and 18 silver and bronze medals were made possible by the technique known as "double doping." During the summer of 2001 I found the only known plan for this program. It was called the "Manual for the Use of Performance-Enhancing Drugs in the 1980 Olympics." This secret plan was for wrestlers and shows how they tested for a decrease of the level of steroids in the urine sample. Using the observations they had made during preparations for the 1979 world championships, they made plans for every athlete who was a medal candidate for the 1980 Games. Even the junior athletes were drugged. The number of candidates seems small only because the specially drugged group is identified; the other 100 elite wrestlers having received "only" anabolics and other drugs during that year. Short rest breaks saved the state money and helped the athletes recover for the next dose.

There is also the case of an East German doctor who tried to stop the doping of athletes. He was employed at the Elite Sport Camp Zinnowitz on the island of Usedom, where he encountered a mandatory doping system he could not accept. So in 1990 he provided information about the organised doping system to the new government of the formerly East German provinces. The new president, Dr Hans Modrow, and the vice-minister of sport, Prof. Dr. Edelfried Buggel, now had an opportunity to read about the legal steroid Oral-Turinabol® and the illegal steroid STS (an experimental drug). To his credit, this physician wrote in a very critical fashion about the health dangers posed by doping: "The drugs had to work quickly and be both inexpensive and effective. That they would damage the health of the athlete was accepted." This letter had no consequences for the doping program because doping was regarded as a necessary strategy. What is more, the very people who were asked to deal with the problem were those responsible for compulsory doping.

Official doping manuals produced by the state confirm that side-effects were well known but kept secret. The files also demonstrate that doping had negative health effects on many women. This detailed knowledge about the consequences of steroid abuse had no effect on the doping program.

The "perfect" integration of drug abuse into the training regimen had consequences for the internal testing system. The record-breaking swimmer Kristin Otto was found to be positive in 1989 as a consequence of the internal drug testing that screened athletes headed for competitions abroad. The sports club to which Kristin Otto belonged doped these girls without their knowledge by calling these treatments nutrition. The experimental anabolic steroids were camouflaged as vitamin pills. In 1989 it was found that Kristin Otto had a very high testosterone level, but she was allowed to travel abroad because the medical staff knew that her testosterone level would not exceed the maximum level allowed by the International Olympic Committee drug-testing program.

The GDR system did not stop this abuse despite the dangers of such high doses. Its alternative to curbing the abuse was research on decreased endogenous hormone production and virilisation. A secret manual described two dangerous side-effects for men and women: inhibition of sperm production as well as gynaecomastia in men, and menstrual-cycle anomalies and virilisation in women.

Compulsory doping also had a strong impact on professional ethics. Doping was practised even as it conflicted with existing laws. The state approved and issued orders in conformity with its secret rules. The sports organisations participated in this "scientific" program, as well. Cryptic and euphemistic terms such as "supportive medications" contributed to diverting attention from the ethical dimension of what was going on. No one took responsibility for the welfare of the athletes.

The medical personnel abetted this system by identifying five allegedly clinical indications that legitimated the prescribing of steroids for athletes. This was, of course, a gimmick, since a condition like exhaustion – designated "deficient catabolic metabolic state" – was experienced by every athlete engaged in high-level training. The doctors justified doping as a necessary form of therapy by expanding the definition of illness as they saw fit. Ethically corrupt medical personnel thus guaranteed that the long-term medical interests of the athletes would not be served.

A research project on the use of hypoxia (the breathing of oxygen-depleted air) began in 1988. This secret and expensive project found that hypoxia training benefited swimmers to a significant degree. Men would swim 1% and women 1.5% faster than under normal conditions. In 1984 the prognosis for all swimming events had been for an improvement of 2%, and without the use of doping. The combination of doping and hypoxia was meant to make East German runners more competitive against Ethiopian athletes. Engineers developed a portable breathing apparatus for this purpose, but the results were not as promising as expected. The technique for combining steroid doping with hypoxia training thus ended rather abruptly in 1984, due to a financial crisis, resistance from athletes, and the departure of the head of the "doping group."

Conclusion

So how unique was the GDR doping program? First, athletes were subjected to compulsory doping because they belonged to special cadres that encouraged a degree of conformity that made resistance almost impossible. Compulsory doping was supervised and financed by the state unimpeded by legal restrictions. The central doping guidelines and plans of the sports federations even regulated the doses taken by their athletes. The Secret Service, the military and the SED guaranteed the supply of drugs. Illegal experimental substances with unknown side-effects were also used. Because athletes already reached threshold levels of doping while still juniors, they could look forward to long careers as drug abusers. Athletic achievement was considered more important than health. At the end of a career the medical data were falsified without the victim's knowledge.

To this day, those athletes who left sport having received false diagnoses of their health problems do not know anything about the medical consequences of the compulsory doping to which they were subjected without their consent.

Which lessons can we draw from the history of state doping in the GDR? First, the GDR invented almost all forms of doping in elite sport that are still being used today, including the abuse of human growth hormone (HGH), plasma expanders (for blood doping), creatine, insulin, opiates, analgesics, and EPO. Second, the supervised use of doping drugs does not reduce the use of the drugs or prevent harm to the athlete's health. This is the most fundamental and verifiable lesson for today's elite sports culture. Third, independent random controls carried out during training minimize the use of doping. Fourth, public discussion of the side-effects of doping also helps to reduce the use of doping drugs.

Compulsory doping created problems for its victims even beyond the medical disorders we have mentioned, including long-term psychological effects such as sex-drive dysfunctions caused by the consumption of anabolic steroids and addictions that arose as surrogates for drug-induced experiences during their athletic careers. The withholding of information from athletes about their own drug consumption led to their drawing false conclusions about the consequences of their own doping regimens. For example, an athlete might say: "I took 'supportive medications' but they did not harm me because there was medical supervision. In the GDR doping wasn't dangerous if you followed the rules." Today's proponents of "medically supervised" doping should consider the medical damage done to East German athletes before proceeding further down this road.

References

Bauersfeld, K.-H./Olek, J./Meissner, H./Hannemann, D./Spanke, J.: Analyse des Einsatzes u. M. [performance-enhancing drugs] in den leichtathletischen Wurf-/ Stossdisziplinen und Versuch trainingsmethodischer Ableitungen und Verallgemeinerungen. DVfL der DDR, Wissenschaftliches Zentrum, ohne Ort [Leipzig] 1973, maschinenschriftlich. [Ex libris B. Berendonk.].

Baur, J./Spitzer, G./Telschow, S: Der DDR-Sport als gesellschaftliches Teilsystem. In: Sportwissenschaft 27 (1997), p. 369-390.

Bette, K.-H./Schimank, U.: Doping im Hochleistungssport. Anpassung durch Abweichung. Frankfurt/Main 1995.

Bette, K.-H./Schimank, U.: Coping mit Doping: Die Sportverbaende im Organisationsstress. In: Sportwissenschaft 26 (1996), p. 357-382.

Delow, A.: Leistungssport und Ideologie – die Vorbereitung der Olympischen Spiele in einem DDR-Sportclub. In: Meyer & Meyer: Sozial- und Zeitgeschichte des Sports 11 (1997) 2, p. 63-81.

Schuhmann, A.: Leistungssport in der DDR – effiziente Ausnahmeerscheinung oder Spiegelbild der Gesellschaft? Unveroeffentlichte Magisterarbeit. Berlin 1997.

Singler, A./Treutlein, G.: Doping im Spitzensport, Sportwissenschaftliche Analysen zur nationalen und internationalen Leistungsentwicklung. Meyer & Meyer: Aachen 2000.

Singler, A./Treutlein, G.: Doping – Analyse und Praevention. Meyer & Meyer: Aachen 2001.

Spitzer, G.: Die DDR-Leistungssportforschung der achtziger Jahre als Subsystem: Thesen zur interdisziplinaeren Systemkritik eines historischen Phaenomens in differenzierungstheoretischer Perspektive. In: Gissel, N. et al. (Hrsg.): Sport als Wissenschaft. Hamburg 1997, p. 151-186.

Spitzer, G.: Der Beitrag von Personen – Stationen des Dopingmissbrauchs durch die Sportspitze der DDR. In: Seppelt, H.-J./Schueck, H. (Hrsg.): Anklage: Kinderdoping. Das Erbe des DDR-Sports. Tenea: Berlin 1999a, p. 97-115.

Spitzer, G.: Spaetschaeden durch Doping bei Sportlern der ehemaligen DDR. In: Mueller-Platz. C. (Red.): Leistungsmanipulation: eine Gefahr fuer unsere Sportler. Sport und Buch Strauss: Koeln 1999b, p. 27-46.

Spitzer, G.: Wie offen war der Verhandlungspartner NOK der DDR? Zur Rolle des MfS in den Beziehungen zum Sport in der Bundesrepublik. In: Grupe, O. (Hrsg.): Einblicke. Aspekte olympischer Erziehung. [Festschrift fuer W. Troeger.] Hofmann: Schorndorf: 1999c, p. 107-112.

Spitzer, G.: Doping in der DDR. Ein historischer Ueberblick zu einer konspirativen Praxis. Genese – Verantwortung – Gefahren. Sport und Buch Strauss: Koeln 1998[1], 2000[2]; Third Edition: April 2004.

Spitzer, G.: Vom Alt-Nazi zum fuehrenden SED-Funktionaer. Neue Fakten zum Leben und Wirken von Sport- und Dopingchef Manfred Ewald. Das falsche Bild vom Widerstandskaempfer wird revidiert. In: Die Welt, 12. Juli 2000.

Spitzer, G.: Manfred Ewald habe "den richtigen hitlerischen Fuehrungstyp verkoerpert". In: Die Welt 13,. Juli 2000.

Spitzer, G.: Auch IAAF-Praesident Paulen stuetzte DDR-Staatsdoping. Stasi-Akten belegen Manfred Ewalds Zynismus In: Die Welt, 14. Juli 2000

Spitzer, G.: Doping in the former GDR. In: Peters, C. et al. (Ed.): Biomedical Side Effects of Doping. Project of the European Union. Bundesinstitut fuer Sportwissenschaft. Sport und Buch Strauss: Koeln 2001a, p. 115-125.

Spitzer, G.: Auswirkungen von Doping bei Frauen. Ethische und ihre Missachtung im DDR-Leistungssport. In: Anders, G./Braun-Laufer, E. (Red.): Grenzen fuer Maedchen und Frauen im Sport. Sport und Buch Strauss: Koeln 2001b, p. 83-100.

Spitzer, G.: Doping with Children. In: Peters, C. et al. (Ed.): Biomedical Side Effects of Doping. Project of the European Union. Bundesinstitut fuer Sportwissenschaft. Sport und Buch Strauss: Koeln 2001c, p. 127-139.

Spitzer, G.: Doping in der DDR als nachhaltiges Modell. In: Helmut Digel / Hans-Hermann Dickhuth (Hrsg.): Doping im Sport. Ringvorlesung der Universität Tübingen. Attempo: Tuebingen 2002, p. 166-191.

Spitzer, G.: Blutdoping als Domaene im Wintersport. Eine Therapie, die in der DDR der Leistungsmanipulation seit 1972 gebraeuchlich war. In: Neue Zuercher Zeitung, 16. Maerz 2002c.

Spitzer, G.: "Sicherungsvorgang Sport". Das Ministerium für Staatssicherheit und der DDR-Spitzensport. Schriftenreihe des Bundesinstituts fuer Sportwissenschaft Band 97. Hofmann: Schorndorf 2004b (Control of GDR sports by the secret State security; in print for June 2004, German language, 648 pages; 200 pages documents).

Spitzer, G. (Ed.): European Doping. London 2004a (forthcoming).

Spitzer, G. et al. (Hrsg.): Schluesseldokumente zum DDR-Sport. Ein sporthistorischer Ueberblick in Originalquellen. Meyer & Meyer: Aachen 1998a, 334 p.

Spitzer, G./Treutlein, G.: DSB-Mann verharmlost Doping. In: Sueddeutsche Zeitung, 27. November 1998.

Spitzer, G./Treutlein, G.: Arbeitsgruppe II: Eine Schluesselposition – Die Rolle des Trainers im Spannungsfeld unterschiedlicher Erwartungen. In: Bundeszentrale fuer gesundheitliche Aufklaerung BZgA

(Hrsg.): Suchtpraevention im Sportverein. Erfahrungen, Moeglichkeiten und Perspektiven fuer die Zukunft. Koeln 2001, p. 84-89 und 90-93.

Teichler, H.J./Reinartz, K. (Hrsg.): Das Leistungssportsystem der DDR in den 80er Jahren und im Prozess der Wende. Schriftenreihe des Bundesinstituts fuer Sportwissenschaft Band 96. Hofmann: Schorndorf 1999.

Waddington, I.: The Development of Doping and Doping Control in Britain. In: Spitzer, G. (Ed.): European Doping. London 2004 (forthcoming).

Notes

1 See the following articles in "Die Welt": "Vom Alt-Nazi zum fuehrenden SED-Funktionaer. Neue Fakten zum Leben und Wirken von Sport- und Dopingchef Manfred Ewald. Das falsche Bild vom Widerstandskaempfer wird revidiert." In: "Die Welt" 12. Juli 2000. Or: Manfred Ewald "incarnated the correct leadership style based on Hitler." In: "Die Welt" 13. Juli 2000. Or: "Auch IAAF-Praesident Paulen stuetzte DDR-Staatsdoping. Stasi-Akten belegen Manfred Ewalds Zynismus." In: Die Welt 14. Juli 2000. Or: "Berliner Dopingprozess vor neuer Ausgangslage? DDR-Sportchef Manfred Ewald als Nazi entlarvt." In: Neue Zuercher Zeitung 24. Mai 2000.

2 The most recent scholarly literature is: Bette/Schimank, Singler/Treutlein, Spitzer. The methods used were document analyses, content analyses, and interviews.

3 Cf. Spitzer, Giselher: "Sicherungsvorgang Sport". Das Ministerium für Staatssicherheit und der DDR-Spitzensport. Schriftenreihe des Bundesinstituts für Sportwissenschaft Band 97 (Control of GDR sports by the secret State security; forthcoming in Summer 2003, in German, 893 pages, 53 documents).

CHAPTER 9

THE ANTI-DOPING CAMPAIGN – FAREWELL TO THE IDEALS OF MODERNITY?

Verner Møller

There is a long tradition of self-governance within Western sport. The founder of the modern Olympic Games, Pierre de Coubertin, made a point of insisting that sport and politics should be preserved as separate realms. He thus encouraged the now widespread view that sport constitutes an ideal world that is highly vulnerable to political interference. However, as sport's popularity has grown, the idea that sport and politics should be kept apart has become more difficult to maintain. The expansion of the mass media has opened up new opportunities for converting athletic superiority into national prestige, and many nations have embraced this strategy. The exploitation of sport by Eastern European countries as a weapon in the ideological struggle against the capitalist societies was seen in the West as a contemptible corruption of the ideals of sport. Western observers attributed the disproportionate harvest of Olympic medals by the Eastern bloc to their violations of the rules of amateurism. The Eastern bloc athletic stars were so-called state amateurs, people who held pro forma jobs, in the army for instance, but who were able to live and train as full-time professional athletes. This form of cheating was seen as additional evidence that the Communist regimes rejected the bourgeois ideals of enlightenment and freedom that constituted the foundation of the Western ethos. The fall of the Berlin Wall and the opening of the Stasi archives provided the free world with essential insights into the origins of the East German "sports miracle." Suspicions about Communism's unscrupulous exploitation of athletes turned out to be entirely justified.

While the Cold War was still underway, the West found it difficult to accept being outdone by the Eastern European countries while the whole world was looking. For this reason the Western countries adopted a more militant sports strategy and invested heavily in their various sports organisations, hoping that better economic circumstances could make their athletes better able to compete. The primary responsibility for administering these funds was left to the sports organisations themselves. Despite the political interest in – not to mention the necessity of – matching the massive Eastern European investment in sport, direct political intervention in sports policy was avoided. In effect, the Western countries waged the ideological struggle on the field of sport in conformity with the bourgeois ideals of freedom on which capitalism is based. These societies created favorable conditions for sport, but the primary impetus remained the ambition of the individual athlete.

In 1998, almost a decade after the end of the Cold War, the time-honoured tradition of self-administration in European sport was history. Acting on the orders of the French minister for youth and sport, Marie-George Buffet, the authorities launched a raid on the world's greatest cycling event, the Tour de France. This intervention produced revelations about doping practices on a scale that made it clear to the sporting public that doping was a systematic and integral part of professional cycling. The minister's initiative was clearly prompted by a sincere concern about the health of the athletes – a concern that, judging from the media coverage, resonated widely throughout French society. These doping revelations also led to the establishment of the global anti-doping agency known as WADA. Although set up as an independent organisation, WADA is subject to political pressure. This political vulnerability creates special difficulties for sports federations, such as the International Cycling Federation (UCI), which is not eager to see a repeat of the 1998 Tour de France scandal, and which is also not particularly happy about giving up any of its powers to WADA.

WADA's objective is to create a doping-free sport culture in several ways. It disseminates information about the harmful effects of doping, promotes the ideal of fair play, and strengthens doping controls while harmonising sanctions against athletes who dope. To the extent that the use of some doping drugs involves serious health risks for the athletes, there is good reason to applaud this anti-doping initiative. But there is also reason for skepticism. Because the clearly strong (political) will to promote the cause of good is inseparable from a correspondingly strong resolve to wage a campaign against evil, and this implacable position leaves no room for tolerance of any kind. On the contrary, it encourages a no-holds-barred approach in an area where it might be wiser to proceed in a less categorical fashion. One may hold the view that political authorities and sports organisations have been too restrained in their policies and even tolerant of athletes' use of doping drugs, with the result that the problem has spun out of control. However, there are reasons to believe this is not the case. For example, the chairman of Anti Doping Denmark, Bengt Saltin, began an article in *Politiken* as follows:

> Myths arise easily and are difficult to dispel, even in the presence of the strongest counter-arguments. There is a widespread misunderstanding to the effect that virtually all elite athletes dope themselves. The fact is that it may be closer to one percent of the very best elite athletes, and in many sports it is more like zero percent. This is the case, not just here in Denmark, but around the world. The evidence is clear! (Saltin 2002).

Saltin finds one piece of evidence in the world of professional cycling:

> The International Cycling Union (UCI) started its "clean-up operation" in 2000 and continued it in 2001. A survey of the 600 best riders who were screened by means of blood testing in the spring of 2001 showed that about 60 of them may have used EPO. These riders were subjected to further testing, and six of them turned up positive, five of whom were later sanctioned. The indications, therefore, are that about one percent were involved in doping in international cycling during the spring of 2001. (Saltin 2002).

When an anti-doping expert of Bengt Saltin's calibre treats "the myth of the doped elite" in this fashion, we are likely to be surprised. On the one hand, he asserts that the sports organisations are doing a fine job of keeping their own houses in order. Self-governance seems to be working. Even the UCI, its tarnished reputation notwithstanding, seems to be capable of handling these problems when it chooses to pay attention to them. This witness claims that the doping problem is almost negligible. According to Saltin, we are only talking about one percent of the athletes in the most affected sports. From this perspective the WADA initiative seems superfluous, the political intervention appears unnecessary, and the campaign against doping is overfunded. In summary, Saltin's account provides a basis for skepticism and further reflection on the entire issue, even if he has too much confidence in drug testing.[1] Doping control is thus no longer an innocent incursion into sport. The time is past when drug-testing simply required an athlete to produce a urine sample after competing – a practice which is, when one thinks about it, quite bizarre in itself. Now the athletes are also required to provide blood samples on demand. As a result of the "necessary" out-of-competition doping controls, the athletes are obligated to report where they are at all times. An even more recent concept in the anti-doping campaign is the so-called "athlete's passport," aimed at making possible an eventual testing procedure for gene doping. The idea here is that athletes undergo a physical examination that yields baseline physiological data, such that deviations from these norms can serve as indirect proof of doping. In other words, the athletes are subjected to an examination that is more comprehensive than anything we know of from any other social sector – so far.

The disproportion between the actual dimensions of the doping problem and the effort being made to eliminate it suggests there are other factors driving the anti-doping campaign apart from athletes' health and the image of sport. The thoughts that follow reflect my suspicion that the anti-doping campaign is fundamentally a symptom of something quite different, namely, a growing lack of confidence in and an unease about the very project of modernity itself. The modern ideal of freedom has opened the world up to strong individual wills that contend with each other and produce an impression of disorder and chaos. This perception has clearly encouraged the mobilizing of a reactionary will to impose order that is exerting pressure on bourgeois legal principles and ideals of freedom.

Anecdotal evidence

A striking example of this pressure was on display at an international conference for critical sports journalists that was held at DGI-byen in Copenhagen in November 2000. One of the themes of the conference was doping, and the presentation by the journalists Olav Skaaning Andersen and Niels Christian Jung, on their prize-winning TV-documentary "The Price of Silence," was a prime attraction. Andersen and Jung showed clips from the program which strongly suggested that, throughout the 1990s, the Danish rider Bjarne Riis used the performance-enhancing drug EPO, thereby implying that his victory in the 1996 Tour de France was achieved through the use of illicit drugs. They described how they gained access to hotel rooms after the riders had left them and how they had removed the contents of their waste baskets before the cleaning personnel arrived.

There are serious questions to be raised about this sort of procedure, wheather the ends justifies the means, yet these questions were not raised on this occasion. The audience, which was made up primarily of journalists, quietly accepted the premise that the ends justified the means. In these waste baskets Andersen and Jung had found hypodermic needles and traces of drugs. Analyses of these samples revealed that they were doping drugs, including EPO. Suffice it to say that "The Price of Silence" did not serve well the reputations of the accused. In fact, the program itself amounted to convicting them in the most public way possible.

When the time for questions arrived I asked the two journalists whether in the course of their ransacking they had come up with any material that could prove that Riis had been doped – the sort of evidence they thought might stand up in a court of law. This question called forth an interesting reaction. Scarcely a moment had passed after Skaaning Andersen acknowledged that they had nothing of the kind, when one of the world's leading doping researchers launched into a passionate defence of Andersen and Jung's initiative and proclaimed the existence of masses of "anecdotal evidence," at which point applause erupted throughout the room.

This demonstrative support for anecdotal evidence as a basis for hanging suspected athletes out to dry in public is interesting because it implies the acceptance of diminished legal rights for athletes in the service of the virtuous campaign against doping. One might point out, of course, that what Andersen and Jung did to Riis has nothing to do with legal rights. Riis was never convicted or even indicted. And even if things looked bad for another Danish cycling star, Bo Hamburger, when he tested positive for EPO in 2001, he was eventually exonerated when one of the two B-samples turned out to be negative. His acquittal occurred despite the fact that the chairman of Anti Doping Denmark, Bengt Saltin, made it clear to the public that Hamburger was guilty. According to the medical experts, even the negative test result was positive, since this sample too deviated significantly from the norm. What saved Hamburger was simply the fact that the margin of uncertainty was too wide to ensure that innocent athletes would not be convicted as a result of the test. In accordance with the ideals of a modern society that is founded upon the rule of law, this doubt benefited the accused.

And yet there is reason for concern. For the public pillorying of those who are suspected of doping is, unmistakably, punishment. Bo Hamburger was dismissed from his CSC-World Online team and banned for life from the national team by the Danish Cycling Federation (DCU). The DCU justified this exclusion by claiming that Hamburger had violated its ethical standards. While the precise nature of these rules remains unclear, the Hamburger affair suggests that a rider has broken them the moment he is suspected of doping and has thus (involuntarily) brought cycling into disrepute. After Hamburger's exoneration by the legal system, the cycling federation argued repeatedly that his exclusion was justified by the fact that he could not account for the unusually high red-blood cell levels indicated by the drug test he had taken. The DCU seems to have opted for a juridical practice comparable to that of the medieval inquisition that condemned those who could not clear themselves of suspicion.

Some people will feel that none of this constitutes reason for concern. It is true that being condemned in the court of public opinion involves emotional and economic costs for the athlete who is under suspicion; but the legal process is based on rules, and after his acquittal the accused can make up his losses by filing a claim for damages. Some may find this result reassuring. Closer analysis will demonstrate, however, that what we are currently witnessing within the world of sport may be a portent of a more general departure from the ideals on which the modern world is based.

The anti-doping campaign's assault on the ideals of the modern world

An essential characteristic of the modern world is that we do not rely on signs and portents. The modern world is founded instead on a confidence in human reason and judgement, and its ideal human type is the citizen who is free, autonomous, and enlightened. But the dismay occasioned by athletes' doping practices is clearly so great that in certain moments of passion people are prepared to discard this ideal as though it did not matter.

It was the very foundation of modernity, rationality itself, that was thrown overboard during the doping furor that erupted after the doping revelations resulting from the 1998 Tour de France. This debate was marked above all by spontaneous condemnations of the athletes involved. The disapproval of the opinion-leaders was summed up in the claim that any use of doping was indiscriminately classified as doping abuse. Language pronounced its own moral condemnation of this behaviour. The most pessimistic voices in this choir did not hesitate to predict the imminent death of sport itself unless quick and effective action were taken against the evil that was threatening its survival. The rhetoric bore witness to an almost religious engagement in the anti-doping struggle, and one must wonder what it was in the doping revelations that produced such violent feelings.

It is worth keeping in mind that the doping practices we find in the context of the Tour de France are different in kind from the compulsory doping that was practised in the former East Germany, where children and adolescents, without their knowledge or that of their parents, were subjected to medically dangerous doping regimens. It is obvious that we should condemn compulsory doping, whether it is innocent children, dogs or horses who are subjected to this kind of treatment.

On the other hand, if we consider the voluntary use of doping drugs in light of the Enlightenment ideal of unprejudiced reason, we will find no solid foundation for condemning such practices. One is forced to acknowledge that the widespread disapproval of elite athletes' use of doping is basically a matter of taste. The only real justification the opponent of doping can offer is that he just doesn't like it.

This is obviously a poor argument to use against athletes' use of doping drugs. It is, therefore, tempting to assert that athletes bear a special responsibility by invoking their value as ideal models. Thus if one claims that athletes due to their position as role models bear a responsibility beyond that of every individual, wheather it be as consumers of tobaccos, injectable drugs, or junk food, it would then appear that a major critique of this position has been founded. Founded on the fact that in this scenario the use of drugs is dangerous, not only for the athletes, but also for the young people who look up to them. For this reason, the argument that athletes have an obligation to be role models has an unquestionable appeal. Upon closer inspection, however, this idea turns out to be quite problematic. First of all, athletes have no legal obligation to act as role models. Those who want to claim that athletes ought to be on call for this purpose are, given the absence of any compelling rationale, simply off base. This is a matter of taste, and the claim that athletes' symbolic value confers on them a responsibility of this kind is actually no more than an attempt to endow an arbitrary wish with the authority of a valid argument. In addition, if it really were the case that athletes had a formal responsibility as public figures, their obligation to assume responsibility as role models would not extend beyond their behavior in public. In that sense, they could not publicly allow themselves to have unsafe sex, or smoke, or eat fast food, or drink beer or dope themselves. However, what they did at home would have to be treated as a private matter. Athletes often have problems living up to their status as role models when it comes to alcohol, smoking, sex and food. But when athletes dope themselves, they always carefully try to prevent it from being publicly exposed. They sometimes even nurture their status as public role models, by claiming their disrespect toward doping users, although this strategy can have unintended consequences. The sprinter Linford Christie and the professional cyclist Jan Ullrich are only two of many athletes who have made a point of publicly distancing themselves from the use of doping drugs – until they tested positive for the use of drugs. And even when they were caught, they came up with all sorts of alibis to try to cover up their use of doping drugs thereby giving their fans reason to believe that, at least as far as doping is concerned, they are as innocent as angels. To be sure, one may try to hold onto the role-modeling argument by maintaining that what one says ought to correspond to what one does, that one ought to live up to one's responsibility. But if we make this a general law for public figures, then it soon becomes clear that this would require a very thorough purge – so thorough, in fact, that it is doubtful any public figures would be left to serve as role-models. The number of politicians, artists and other celebrities who have behaved in ways that, euphemistically speaking, can be described as less than exemplary, is legion. In this context it is worth noting that the immoral and transgressive behavior of these people often contributes in a positive fashion to their images and actually increases their popularity. This could indicate that sports icons setting bad examples for young people is not really the problem. Clearly, nor, it is the problem with sports people that they are promiscuous, alcoholics, or violent, but rather that they allow themselves to take full advantage of the performance-enhancing medical techniques that are a product of modernity. A growing skepticism toward modernity, however, has made it increasingly difficult for late modern people to reconcile themselves with these medical practices. All this should be enough to show that the value of athletes as anti-doping role models has been grossly overrated.

Another problem with which the campaign against doping must reckon is that doping is not a problem *within* sport but rather a problem *of* sport. The frequently heard argument that this campaign protects sport is thus not tenable. In what follows, I will elaborate on this argument before suggesting why doping today provokes such massive resistance.

The essence of sport

My primary assertion is that there is no valid argument against doping that is not at the same time an argument against sport itself. In other words, there is no basis for arguing that athletes' use of doping violates the principles of sport. On the contrary, there is good reason to argue that doping is quite simply a consequence of sport itself.

The principle of sport is best expressed in the Olympic motto: Faster, higher, stronger. Sport's driving force is in its essence the will to achieve victory. If a football player does not want to win, then why should he expose himself to the brutal tackling game and the risks it involves. If the cyclist does not want to win, then why not just let his opponents go when they set an unforgiving pace and the race becomes a brutal test of endurance.

There are, of course, people who play football without any particular concern about who wins, as well as there are people who ride racing bikes because they find it enjoyable and want to get some excercise. However, these people are recreational types, not athletes. So, on the one hand, we may find it fun to play football or ride racing bikes. Or, on the other, we may simply be lazy and envy the discipline of these recreational types or their desire to take a preventive approach to good health in response to the admonitions of the health authorities. However, only a very few of us will find that sort of thing worth watching. For what we value in sport is the uncompromising engagement – the excitement and intensity that come from the fact that victory means something.

When victory does not matter there is nothing at stake and nothing for spectators to watch except meaningless movement. Only a taste for the absurd aspect of life can make us enjoy watching recreational types exercise. Because their engagement in this activity does not amount to much. The recreational types take their exercise to save themselves, even if there is no danger on the horizon. As spectators we do not see whatever it is these people see inside themselves. We don't see death nipping at their heels. For this reason recreational sport, as seen from the outside, is devoid of excitement.

There is, thus, a profound difference between recreational exercise and sport. Recreational sport has a long-range appeal in that it increases one's chances of preserving good health to a ripe old age. Sport, on the other hand, offers an immediate pay-off in the form of intoxicating experiences that involve presence, excitement and an uncompromising devotion that puts health at risk. To practice sport is to exist in the here and now; to use oneself, develop one's talent and seek success without worrying about the price one will pay in the future. The Danish cyclist Brian Holm, who served as a loyal support-rider for Bjarne Riis on the Deutsche Telekom team when Riis was a champion, illustrates this in a striking way in his book *The Pain – The Joy*:

> A teammate once told me that he wanted to take all the drugs that were necessary for him to become a strong rider and a star. He maintained that he could not care less whether doping shortened his life so that he would not even live to be fifty. All he wanted was to win a big race. (Holm 2002: 110).

That is an extreme attitude. But it would be a serious misunderstanding to call it contrary to the spirit of sport. Seen from the proper perspective, this statement expresses a profound sporting attitude. The point being, as I noted earlier, that the primary force in sport is the will to victory. That is why serious athletes train harder and longer than the recreational athletes who exercise. Because a lot of training can give the athlete an advantage over his opponents. It is for the same reason that athletes seek expert assistance in connection with their training regimens. An incompetent trainer will be quickly dismissed no matter how friendly he is, because it is an advantage to have a competent trainer. The same logic prompts athletes to forsake culinary delights if they are competing in sports where less weight is an advantage.

One of the frequently invoked arguments against doping is that it creates unequal competitive conditions. However, as I have already demonstrated, sport is not a matter of equality but rather of evenly matched opponents. And since an even match involves only a partial equality one of the evenly matched partners will usually have an advantage over the other. This is the position every athlete attempts to achieve by means of intensive training, strict diets, coaching advice and just about anything else. Doping is one consequence of this striving for advantage.

What makes the difference, of course, is that doping is not allowed and therefore counts as cheating. Indeed, we are often told that doping is cheating. This is, however, an invalid claim that can be dispensed with quite easily. Because if the reason that we cannot accept doping is that it is cheating, then the simplest solution would be to allow it. If doping were legalised, then it would no longer be cheating. If someone were to object that this is a sophistical refutation, then there are other ways of demonstrating that this is not the fundamental reason that doping is considered cheating, that it provokes dismay and attracts the attention of politicians. There are, to be sure, many rules in sport – there have to be if sport is going to function at all – but it is also well known that breaking the rules of sport is an integral part of sport itself.

Every free kick in football involves a violation of the rules, and many free kicks are accompanied by warnings. When free kicks are accompanied by more warnings and ever fewer expulsions, gross violations multiply. This means that the infractions that are committed put opponents at significant risk of injury. Cheating that does not endanger opponents is less frowned upon. And there are no sanctions at all if someone succeeds in cheating but is not found out until after the competition.

One of the most famous examples of cheating in sport occurred when Maradona used his hand to score a goal during the soccer World Cup in Mexico City in 1986. This goal put Argentina ahead of England by 1-0 and thus gave Argentina a significant advantage. Yet, despite the clear indications that he had cheated, Maradona was hailed as a world champion at the end of the tournament. The referee had not observed this offence in the heat of the competition, so there was nothing to be done about it. But, the fact that this incident led to no rule change whatsoever shows that breaking the rules, if you are smart enough about it, is an accepted part of the game. Because, as a matter of principle, there is no reason not to decide, that if a player is caught scoring with his hand then he should be banned for two years, even if the violation is only detected after the game. In fact this would demonstrate that the ideal of fair play in sport was taken seriously. At the same time, however, there are many examples which demonstrate that fair play is not the alpha and omega of sport. Concepts such as fair play and the spirit of sport are a linguistic sugar-coating that is applied to the bitter pill of sport for the purpose of reassuring sponsors, officials who do the funding, and others who cannot reconcile themselves to the fact that sport is what it is.

Sport as character-building

There is a long tradition telling us about the edifying and character-building effects of sport. Even as sportive realities demonstrate time and time again that the idea of sport as a venue of character-building and health is no more than dreams and suppositions, the desperate struggle to hold on to the idea of the pedagogical qualities of sport continues unabated. The problem is that the real qualities of sport are not the ones we usually hear about.

The contradiction between the after-dinner speeches and the reality of sport was already clear at the 1908 Olympic Games. It was here that bishop Talbot spoke in St. Paul's Cathedral and pronounced the immortal words: "In these Olympiads, the important thing is not winning, but taking part" (Coubertin 2000: 587). No modern marketing expert could have formulated the Olympic ideology better than that, and Coubertin quickly made these words his own in his famous speech during these Games, adding: "The important thing in life is not victory, but struggle: the essential is not to conquer, but to fight well" (Coubertin 2000: 587). Here Coubertin emphasizes the pedagogical mission of the Olympic Games.

That the pedagogical ideal embraced by the bishop and the Olympic statesman coincided neither with the athletes' disposition nor with the essence of Olympic sport became clear during the dramatic conclusion of the marathon. The runner who was leading in the race, Dorando Pietri, collapsed just before the finish line and had to be dragged the rest of the way by eager helpers who felt compassion for the totally exhausted athlete. While underway he had fortified himself with strychnine, and in his eagerness to win he had come close to running himself to death. This episode closely paralleled another drama that had taken place at the St. Louis Olympic Games four years earlier, when the winner of the marathon, Thomas Hicks, had used strychnine to boost his performance. He managed to reach the finish line under his own powers but then collapsed and had to be resuscitated.

All of this suggests that long before the Games were appropriated as a battlefield for great-power politics, and before commercialisation had turned winning into a lucrative business, the pedagogical ideal that rejected winning at any price was already being contradicted by the actual practice of Olympic sport. There is, in fact, every reason to believe that, from the very beginning, sport has stimulated sheer ambition to such a degree that the idea that winning is not the most important goal has never taken root apart from in after-dinner speeches about sport as an educational project.

The real motive force of sport: the will to win has, however, become controversial. To be sure, Dorando Pietri was disqualified after he was helped over the finish line, because he had received inappropriate assistance, but he was not reproached for his uncompromising effort. It was obvious that he could not be proclaimed the victor, but the next day he received a remarkable consolation prize when Queen Alexandra awarded him a gold cup for his heroic deed.

Athletes' use of stimulating drugs was not regarded as a problem at that time. This was not because the use of drugs was unusual or unknown. Within the cycling milieu in particular, experimentation with performance-enhancing drugs was underway throughout the second half of the nineteenth century. It would seem that stimulating drugs were as much a part of the sport as the bicycle itself. The debilitating six-day races and the road races that covered enormous distances prompted the riders to seek out methods that could increase their endurance, and it was found that the so-called speedball, a mixture of heroin and cocaine, was an effective stimulant. Other techniques included sugar cubes soaked in ether, caffeine pills, strychnine and, by the middle of the twentieth century, amphetamines.

It was not until about 1960, when the Danish rider Knud Enemark Jensen died during the Rome Olympic Games, that doping came to be seen as a serious problem. His death prompted the Council of Europe to issue a resolution against doping in 1963. Systematic doping controls were first implemented at the 1968 Mexico City Olympic Games. In the meantime, cycling authorities had begun to outlaw the use of certain drugs and to undertake sporadic drug-testing.

During the 1967 Tour de France, the English rider Tom Simpson died during the televised ascent of Mont Ventoux; his bloodstream found full of amphetamines. While this was bad publicity for cycling, the reactions it provoked were not nearly as violent as those that accompanied the Festina scandal of 1998. Only a year after Simpson's death, the most successful professional rider of all time, Eddy Merckx, was caught doping at the Giro d'Italia race. Given Simpson's high-profile death, one might have thought that Merckx would be dragged down from the victory stand, but this is not what happened. On the contrary, the Belgian government intervened in the matter by defending the reputation of their star cyclist and by threatening to break off all diplomatic relations with Italy if the Italian government did not conduct a thorough investigation of the circumstances surrounding the outrageous doping accusations that were being directed at their national hero. The Belgian government's reaction demonstrates how different the climate of opinion regarding doping was as compared with today.

This difference is also evident in the fact that a monument to Tom Simpson was erected on Mont Ventoux. It is true that the Simpson tragedy gave rise to some criticism; the French media, for example, sowed doubts about his ethical standards. This prompted France's greatest cyclist of this era, the five-time Tour de France winner Jacques Anquetil, to offer a controversial defence of the Englishman. Anquetil argued that Simpson's behaviour was hardly exceptional; on the contrary, all of the riders were doping themselves.

That year Anquetil had set a new record for the one-hour time trial. By this time, however, the UCI had introduced doping controls, and when Anquetil refused to be drug-tested his record was not recognised. Still, Anquetil remained absolutely resolute, insisting that the riders were free and autonomous people and that doping was their own business. As far as he was concerned, the officious paternalism represented by drug testing had no place in professional cycling.

Today many would argue that this is a rash and indefensible point of view. Yet this position is entirely consistent with the ideals that appear in Immanuel Kant's 1783 text "What is Enlightenment?" where he writes:

> Enlightenment is man's release from his self-incurred tutelage. Tutelage is man's inability to make use of his understanding without direction from another. Self-incurred is this

tutelage when its cause lies not in lack of reason but in lack of resolution and courage to use it without direction from another. "Have courage to use your own reason!" – that is the motto of enlightenment. (Kant 1995: 83)

The most determined opponents of doping are likely to resent the spectacle of Kant, this spiritual beacon of Enlightenment thought, being (mis)used to support Anquetil's point of view. They might even assert that Anquetil's early death, due to blood clots in his lungs and to stomach cancer, shows that he was unable to make good use of his rational faculties, and that authorities capable of making rational judgements should have imposed limits on him. As impressive as this argument may seem, it is fundamentally weak as long as it does not address the idea that every autonomous person has the right to manage his own life as he sees fit, so long as he does not abridge the rights of others to do the same. Even if a tendency toward paternalism is becoming evident in more and more areas of modern society, I am not aware of any opponents of doping who have publicly called for the establishment of a paternalistic social order to put an end to doping. For this reason, the most powerful objection against Anquetil's position – that he was unaware of the long-term consequences of his health-endangering behavior and therefore lacked the qualifications to make that decision – remains unconvincing. This argument is acceptable only if one is prepared to live without any defence against a paternalist hegemony. For only in a very few situations do we possess the kind of knowledge that can assure us that the decisions we make now will serve us well in the long run. It seems to be an unavoidable condition for free human beings that they must take chances and run risks in order to achieve their ambitions and goals. For outsiders, and perhaps in retrospect, these goals may appear to be arbitrary, uninteresting or even life-threatening. However, this perspective cannot restrain the person who regards the achievement of that goal as essential to his own life. Moreover, there is nothing that indicates that Anquetil ever regretted the way of life that was so hard on him. On his death bed his capacity for gallows humor became evident when he joked with his old rival, the eternal runner-up Raymond Poulidor and "triumphantly" told him that "once again you are going to be number two" (Brunel 1995).

Nevertheless, a frequently repeated argument against doping is that it is not a free choice for ambitious athletes as they begin to dope themselves when they are immature and are unable to imagine the long-term consequences of their decisions. Those who are *de jure* autonomous are thus rendered *de facto* unautonomous. The implicit message here is that people today are regarded as mature only when they no longer use their rational faculties to accomplish their own goals and have adopted the prevailing and authoritative norms that define what constitutes a healthy, good and sensible life.

The fear of modernity

When Kant talks about having the courage to use one's reason independent of others' directives, he is addressing the motive force that animates the dynamism and progress so characteristic of the modern world. With this in mind it becomes easy to understand why doping has flourished to the degree that it has in cycling. For cycling is the first genuinely modern sport, in that its birth coincided with the invention of a machine. As such, the bicycle is quite simply a product of modernity and was both a triumph for – and a contribution to – optimism about progress. The bicycle expanded the territory of every human life and became thereby a symbol of freedom, independence and of undreamed human possibilities. Indeed, cycling came into existence along with the modern medical research of which the most effective doping drugs are a direct result.

For much of the twentieth century there prevailed a widespread confidence in science and a belief that human potential would develop along with scientific progress. Science in general, and medical science in particular, were generally regarded as inherently good. In the course of time this view has given way to a rather different view of what science portends.

Up until about 1950 the products of medical research were seen as solutions to human problems. Today, however, this research is greeted more skeptically. Even as medical science has developed an impressive array of treatments for disease, it has become clear that medical therapies involve both limits and costs. For this reason it is no longer possible, as it once was during the first phase of modernity, to preserve a naïve belief in science as the way to eternal life and paradise on earth. As science has become more effective and produced revolutionary discoveries, the dark side of this process has become clear.

This process of disillusionment has sowed doubts about both science and the idea of progress itself. The jogging craze of the 1970s and the aerobics and fitness boom of the 1980s can be seen as marking the end of an era during which people dared to rely on science as a form of salvation in the event they encountered health problems. It became fashionable during the 1970s to make regular exercise a part of one's personal lifestyle. But the underlying motive of this behaviour was a growing scepticism about modernity itself. Rather than fearing hunger and hardship, we confront the diseases of civilisation. As our confidence in science as salvation diminishes, our interest in health, as expressed in the shift from treatment to prevention, continues to grow. Health is no longer taken for granted; it has become, instead, a holy blessing. One consequence of this transition is that our original fear of death is transformed (ironically) into a fear of life.

The health argument has also played a central role in the doping debate, even if health as an argument against doping is no more convincing than the others that have been proposed. This is not because there is no satisfactory definition of health. If, for example, one chooses to define health as the *absence of disease*, then doping is not unhealthy as long as it does not make you sick. One might choose instead to invoke the philosopher Steen Wackerhausen's open concept of health, which states that health is the ability to achieve one's genuine and realistic goals under the conditions life happens to provide (Wackerhausen 1994: 49). If we apply this definition, then Bjarne Riis was healthier in 1996, when he fulfilled his genuine and realistic goal of winning the Tour de France, than he was during his previous (and far less successful) racing seasons. And this despite the fact that during the year he won he was dubbed Mr. 60 Percent, a nickname that referred to what was alleged to be an abnormally high hematocrit.

But even if one takes a common-sense understanding of health as one's point of departure, the health argument remains useless. For if sport's legitimacy rests on the premise that it is healthy, then many forms of elite sport should be forbidden, with or without doping, since they cause serious injuries and are unhealthy in other respects. The fact that elite sport puts health at risk is repressed at the same time that it is stubbornly asserted that sport is and ought to be healthy. Torn ligaments, broken bones, fatal crashes and eating disorders are always treated as accidents and never as logical consequences of the pressure that sport exerts on the human physique. So the doping phenomenon cannot be condemned as an unhealthy deviation from the healthy practices of sport.

Thus there is, reason to believe that doping provokes horror and indignation above all because it expresses open disdain for the sacred ideal of health. The very idea that someone would use a hypodermic needle to win an athletic competition is regarded as a form of blasphemy. And the worst thing of all is that courageous people – in this case the doping sinners – take their health for granted. They do not treat health as something sacred but go so far as to show it a reckless disregard. The conflict of interest between the righteous defenders of health and the infidel athletes is thus clear. The infidels – or modernists – use sport for the purpose of confronting the tragic conditions of an impermanent life. They invest their health in the hope of creating for themselves a name and a career, so that their finite lives do not simply pass away, meaningless and unobserved. They try, that is, not to lie about the reality of death by preserving their health. It is no wonder this frightens those who see health as the meaning of existence and who believe that they can secure themselves against sickness and premature death by adopting the right kinds of health behaviours.

The manner in which the doping debate has been carried out since 1998 is reason enough to fear that the modern epoch is in the process of expiring. When one hears proposals for lifetime bans for doping offences; when even the Danish Cycling Federation refuses every compromise with athletes who, like Claus Michael Møller, have violated the doping rules but have served out their penalties; and when the same federation excommunicates Bo Hamburger, despite his exoneration in accordance with the legal rules of the game – at this point we can assume that, at least within the sports world, we are leaving behind modernity's ideals of freedom in favour of a moral practice and a conception of the law modelled after medieval practices. This gives us every reason to hope that sport is not, as it is often claimed to be, a reflection of society. Despite the growing paternalism in many areas of society, it would appear that there are still reasons for hope. Take, for example, the newspaper advertisement for Viagra that the Pfizer pharmaceutical company sponsored during the 2002 football World Cup matches. In this advertisement the company makes surprising use of the football icon Pele, who in this context is sanctioning the use of a performance-enhancing drug for those who have been unable to live up to certain expectations and previous performances. Yet no one issued a peep of protest about this ad. This silence is worth thinking about. It may also serve as a source of comfort for those who watch with trepidation as paternalism continues its march through the world of sport, which is now prepared to treat every elite athlete as a potential criminal.

References

Berendonk, Brigitte (1991): *Doping-Dokumente: Von der Forschung zum Betrug*, Berlin, Rowolth.

Brunel, Philippe (1996): *An Intimate Portrait of The Tour de France – Masters and Slaves of the Road*, Colorado, Buonpane Publications.

Coubertin, Pierre de (2000): *Olympism – Selected Writings*, Lausanne, International Olympic Committee.

Hoberman, John (1992): *Mortal Engines – The Science of Performance and the Dehumanization of Sport*, New York, Free Press.

 – "A Pharmacy on Wheels" in Verner Møller og John Nauright eds.: *The Essence of Sport*, Odense, University of Southern Denmark Press.

Holm, Brian (2002): *Smerten Glæden – Erindringer fra et liv på cykel*, København, Hovedland.

Kant, Immanuel (1995/1959): Foundations of the Metaphysics of Morals and What is Enlightenment?, Translated, with an introduction, by Lewis White Beck, Library of Liberal Arts, Prentice Hall, New Jersey.

Møller, Verner (1999): *Dopingdjævlen*, København, Gyldendal.

 – (2003): "What is Sport: Outline to a Redefinition" in Verner Møller og John Nauright eds.: *The Essence of Sport*, Odense, University of Southern Denmark Press.

 – "Cykelsport og fremskridtsoptimisme" i *Idrætshistorisk årbog 2001*, Odense, Syddansk Universitetsforlag.

Nilsson, Pea (1982): Maratonboken, Stockholm, Manus Förlag.

Rabenstein, Rüdiger (1991): *Radsport und Gesellschaft – Ihre sozialgeschichtlichen Zusammenhänge in der Zeit von 1867 bis 1914*, Hildesheim, Weidmann Verlag.

Saltin, Bengt (2002): "Myten om den dopede atlet", *Politiken* 7. april.

Spitzer, Giselher (1998): Doping in DDR. Ein historischer Überblick zu einer konspirativer Praxis, Köln Bundesinstitut für Sportswissenschaft.

Wackerhausen, Steen (1994): "Et åbent sundhedsbegreb – mellem fundamentalisme og relativisme" i Uffe Juul Jensen og Peter Fuur Andersen red.: *Sundhedsbegreber – filosofi og praksis*, Århus, Philosofia.

Notes

1 It is also difficult to imagine that Saltin is really as confident as his article would have us believe. For he can hardly be unaware of how athletic performances have been developing in recent years. A simple comparison of the average speeds at which the Tour de France has been ridden shows that this measure of performance did not decline after the doping revelations of 1998. On the contrary, the 1999 Tour was the fastest ever and not exceeded until the 2003 Tour, which recorded the fastest average speed of all time. If one believes that doping drugs do enhance athletes' performances, then the increase in speed that has occurred in elite cycling is in itself an indication that doping practices have not decreased. One may thus speculate about what it is that prompted Saltin to draw such obviously implausible conclusions from the results of the doping tests. One possibility is that he wants to demonstrate that the anti-doping campaign after 1998 has been a success, and that continuing this initiative is worth the investment that is required. Another possibility is that, by presenting the doping problem as involving only a very small number of cheaters, he wants to propagate the view that sport is worth fighting for. He is, in effect, pursuing an ideological agenda, in that he is attempting to create the foundation for a modern and rational way to push for a hard anti-doping line. The idea that sport possesses an inherent nobility is highly debatable and beyond the scope of this essay. For a more thorough treatment of this subject, see Møller 2003.

CONTRIBUTORS

Karl-Heinrich Bette is Professor of Sociology of Sport at Darmstadt University of Technology. His main academic interests are the sociology of the body, system theory, sociology of elite sports, and the doping issue. He is the author of many books including: *Körperspuren. Zur Semantik und Paradoxie moderner Körperlichkeit*, (1989), *Doping im Leistungssport– sozialwissenschaftlich beobachtet*, (editor) (1994), *International Sociology of Sport: Contemporary Issues*, (1995), *Doping im Hochleistungssport. Anpassung durch Abweichung*, (1995) (together with Uwe Schimank), *Systemtheorie und Sport*, (1999), *Biographische Dynamiken im Hochleistungssport. Möglichkeiten der Dopingprävention im Jugendalter*, (2002) (together with Uwe Schimank et al.).

Alessandro Donati has served for many years as an elite athletics coach, specialising in the sprints and middle-distance races, at the Central School of Sport of C.O.N.I., where he is Professor of Sport. He holds a degree in the science of coaching from the Université Claude Barnard in Lyon, France. At great personal risk to himself he has been a leader in the struggle against doping in Italy since the 1980s. He is author of the book *Campioni senza valore* (Victories Without Value) (1989).

John Hoberman has been active in sports studies for the past 25 years as a scolar and journalist. He is author of *Sport and Political Ideology* (1984), *The Olympic Crisis: Sport, Politics and the Moral Order* (1986), *Mortal Engines: The Science of Performance and the Dehumanization of Sport* (1992), *Darwin's Athletes: How Sport has Damaged Black America and Preserved the Myth of Race* (1997), and *Testosterone Dreams: Rejuvenation, Aphrodisia, Doping* (forthcoming). He is Professor of Germanic Studies at the University of Texas at Austin, Texas, and Visiting Professor at the University of Southern Denmark (Odense).

Barrie Houlihan is Professor at Loughborough University. His research interests include the development of theory to understand domestic and international policy processes for sport. He has a particular interest in the diplomatic use of sport, the politics of the Olympic movement, drug abuse by athletes and the sports development policy. He has undertaken consultancy projects for the Sports Council. He is currently a member of the English Sports Council's working group on sports strategy. His extensive list of publications includes: *Sport and International Politics* (1994), *Sport, Policy and Politics: A Comparative Analysis* (1997), and *Dying to Win: the Development of Anti-doping Policy* (1999).

Patrick Laure is a sociologist and an associated researcher, at the Laboratory of Applied Psychology, University of Reims. His main publications count: *Le dopage* (1995), *Les gélules de la performance* (1997), *Dopage et société* (2000), *L'éthique du dopage* (2002), and (with C. Binsinger) *Détournement de l'usage des médicaments* (2003).

Verner Møller is Associate Professor at the Institute of Sport Science and Clinical Biomechanics, in the Faculty of Health Sciences at the University of Southern Denmark (Odense). He has edited and written books on sports, health and doping, including *Masker og mål: Undersøgelse af vilkår i dansk elite håndbold* (*Masks and Balls: A Study of Elite Handball in Denmark*) (1995), *Sundhed og idræt: Kulturanalyser til indkredsning af sundhedsaspektet i idrætten* (*Health and Sport: Cultural Analysis and Defining the Health Dimension in Sport*) (1999), and *Dopingdjævlen* (*The Doping Devil*) (1999), which is currently being translated into English. His most recent edited book, in collaboration with John Nauright, is *The Essence of Sport* (2003).

Andreas Singler studied sports at the Johannes-Gutenberg-Universität in Mainz where he works as a freelance sports and science journalist. His list of publications includes: *Doping in Spitzensport. Sportwissenschaftliche Analysen zur nationalen und internationalen Leistungsentwicklung* (2000), und *Doping – von der Analyse zur Prävention. Vorbeugung gegen abweichendes Verhalten in soziologischem und pädagogishem Zugang* (2001) (both co-authored by Gerhard Treutlein).

Hans B. Skaset is Professor at Norwegian University of Sport and Physical Education. From the late 1960s he has held central positions in Norwegian sport, with continuous engagement in the anti-doping campaign at national and international levels. Until 2000 he was Director General, at the Department of Sport Policy, in the Norwegian Ministry of Cultural Affairs. He is founder of the international anti-doping organisation IADA.

Giselher W. Spitzer is Privatdozent at the University Potsdam. He has studied history, social science and sport science and his academic interests include Social- and contemporary history of sports, didactics and methodology of the ball-games, health-education and public health. His expertise covers the development and sport science in the GDR, the East German state-sponsored doping program, and transformation processes in the GDR following the collapse of the East German State in 1989/90. He has been active in the prevention of doping in sports in cooperation with German Health organization. His most recent books are: *Schluesseldokumente zum DDR-Sport. Ein sporthistorischer Ueberblick in Originalquellen* (1998), *Doping in der DDR. Ein historischer Ueberblick zu einer konspirativen Praxis. Genese – Verantwortung – Gefahren* (1998), *Fußball und Triathlon* (2004).

Gerhard Treutlein is Professor and head of the Sports Sciences and Sports Pedagogics department of the University of Education of Heidelberg, Germany. His major research interest is the training of teachers and coaches, including the study of teacher-pupil and coach-athlete interaction models. As a former coach of high level athletes and actual responsible for athletics in the German federation of university sports (ADH – since 1972) he also has a long standing interest in the development of doping and the struggle against doping. He is author of several books including: *Sport und Gesellschaft* (1995), *Sport und Sportunterricht in Frankreich und Deutschland* (1994), *Sportwissenschaft in Deutschland und Frankreich* (1997), *Doping im Spitzensport. Sportwissenschaftliche Analysen zur nationalen und internationalen Leistungsentwicklung* (2000) (with Andreas Singler) *Doping – von der Analyse zur Prävention* (2001) (with Andreas Singler), and *Körper, Sport und Religion* (2002).

Ivan Waddington is Visiting Professor at the Norwegian University of Sport and Physical Education, Oslo; at University College Chester UK; and at the Centre for Sports Studies, University College Dublin, Ireland. He has published extensively in the sociology of health and the sociology of sport and much of his work has focused on the interface between health and sport. He is author of *Sport, Health and Drugs* (2000) and a co-author of *Drugs in Sport: The Pressure to Perform* (2002), which is the official policy statement of the British Medical Association on doping in sport. He has also provided expert advice on doping to the European Commission.